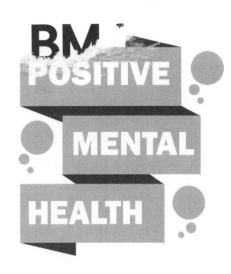

BMA

POSITIVE

MENTAL

HEALTH

SUPPORTING STUDENT MENTAL HEALTH
IN HIGHER EDUCATION

POSITIVE MENTAL HEALTH

This new series of texts presents a modern and comprehensive set of evidence-based strategies for promoting positive mental health in young people. There is a growing prevalence of mental ill-health in the young within a context of funding cuts, strained services and a lack of formal training for teachers and tutors. The series recognises the complexity of the issues involved, the vital role that educational professionals play and the current education and health policy frameworks, in order to provide practical guidance backed up by the latest research.

You might also like:

Effective Personal Tutoring in Higher Education by Dave Lochtie, Emily McIntosh, Andrew Stork and Ben Walker, Critical Publishing, 2018. ISBN: 978-1-910391-98-3

Our titles are also available in a range of electronic formats. To order, or for details of our bulk discounts, please go to our website www.criticalpublishing.com or contact our distributor, NBN International, 10 Thornbury Road, Plymouth PL6 7PP, telephone 01752 202301 or email orders@nbninternational.com.

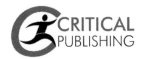

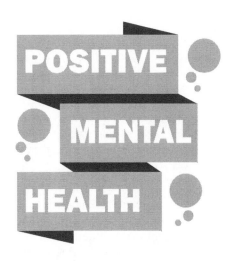

POSITIVE

MENTAL

HEALTH

SUPPORTING STUDENT MENTAL HEALTH

IN HIGHER EDUCATION

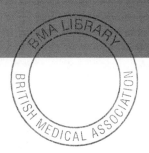

Samuel Stones and Jonathan Glazzard

First published in 2019 by Critical Publishing Ltd

British Library Cataloguing in Publication Data
A CIP record for this book is available from the British Library

ISBN: 978-1-912508-77-8

This book is also available in the following e-book formats:

MOBI ISBN: 978-1-912508-78-5
EPUB ISBN: 978-1-912508-79-2
Adobe e-book ISBN: 978-1-912508-80-8

Cover and text design by Out of House Limited
Project Management by Newgen Publishing UK
Printed and bound in Great Britain by 4edge, Essex

Critical Publishing
3 Connaught Road
St Albans
AL3 5RX

www.criticalpublishing.com

Paper from responsible sources

✚ CONTENTS

✚ MEET THE SERIES EDITOR AND AUTHORS

SAMUEL STONES

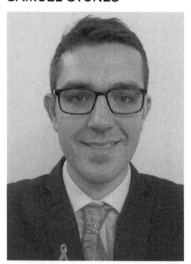

JONATHAN GLAZZARD

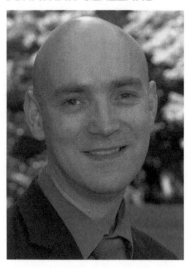

Samuel Stones is an Associate Researcher in the Carnegie School of Education at Leeds Beckett University. His research outputs are linked with the Centre for LGBTQ+ Inclusion in Education and the Carnegie Centre of Excellence for Mental Health in Schools. Samuel's research explores the experiences of teachers who identify as lesbian, gay, bisexual and transgender, with specific emphasis on the impact of sexual orientation on teacher identity and mental health. He also works with initial teacher training students in university and school contexts and is an Associate Leader of maths, computing, economics and business at a secondary school and sixth form college in North Yorkshire.

Jonathan Glazzard is editor for the Positive Mental Health series by Critical Publishing. He has produced an extensive range of books on mental health, special educational needs and disabilities and early reading development. He has also produced many journal articles. Jonathan teaches across all levels on undergraduate, masters and doctoral programmes. He was awarded a National Teaching Fellowship in 2015 for his contribution to teaching in higher education.

+ INTRODUCTION

Headline news in recent months has highlighted the extent of student mental ill-health in the United Kingdom. The media report that an increasing number of students in higher education are experiencing stress, anxiety, depression, self-harm, eating disorders and social and emotional problems. Cases of student suicides have also been reported in the national press.

The massification of higher education in the UK has resulted in an increasingly diverse student population over the past two decades. This has helped universities to advance social justice by transforming students' life chances. Alongside this, the Equality Act (2010) places a legal duty on higher education providers to ensure that students with protected characteristics have equality of opportunity. Mental ill-health can impact detrimentally not only on students' well-being but also on their academic attainment. If higher education institutions do not provide adequate support for students with mental ill-health, there is an increased risk that they will either withdraw from their courses or achieve lower academic and employment outcomes than students who are mentally healthy.

As this book goes to press there are also increasing concerns being raised about the mental health of staff who work in higher education. Concerns have been raised not only about staff workload, but also about a culture of bullying that some staff have reported. If lecturing staff are not mentally healthy, this will impact on the quality of teaching and also on the quality of support that they provide for students. Staff absence does not support a positive student experience.

Going to university is an exciting time for students. It is accompanied by a series of multiple and multidimensional transitions and these can result in mental ill-health if they are not smooth. Students may be moving away from home for the first time. While managing the challenges associated with living independently, students must manage new academic and social transitions. They will form new friendships, develop new interests and be introduced to different models of teaching and assessment to those used within school and college contexts. These transitions can be exciting but also stressful as students learn to navigate them. In this

1

book you will be introduced to theoretical perspectives on transitions into and through higher education and you will find out about how to support students through these.

You will be introduced to specific barriers to learning, participation and achievement experienced by different groups of students. You will learn about your responsibilities as a personal tutor or a lecturer in supporting positive mental health in students. Implications for university leaders and managers are also stated.

The book promotes an institution-wide approach for supporting students' mental health. The elements of this approach are addressed and implications for higher education policies and practices are identified.

Student mental health in higher education is everyone's concern. It is not one person's responsibility. The emphasis on supporting student mental health in institutions needs to focus on all students and not just those students who demonstrate signs of mental ill-health. By adopting an institution-wide approach, universities can create mentally healthy campuses that enable all students to experience a sense of belonging and to thrive.

We hope you enjoy reading this book and find it useful.

Samuel Stones and Jonathan Glazzard

✛ CHAPTER 1

TRANSITIONS INTO HIGHER EDUCATION

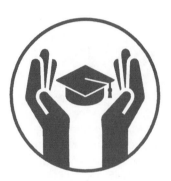

PROFESSIONAL LINKS

This chapter addresses the following:

The Teaching Excellence Framework (TEF) emphasises the need for higher education providers to recruit students from under-represented groups. It also places an emphasis on student retention.

CHAPTER OBJECTIVES

After reading this chapter you will understand:

+ the multiple and multidimensional nature of transition;

+ the role of schools, colleges and universities in supporting student transitions into higher education;

+ the role of induction in supporting transition;

+ how to facilitate smooth transitions through the first year.

INTRODUCTION

Over several years policy initiatives in the United Kingdom have focused on widening participation in higher education. The focus on increasing the numbers of students from diverse backgrounds in higher education has drawn attention to the need for institutions to improve student engagement and retention (Gale and Parker, 2014). Consequently, there is a need to give greater attention to ways in which higher education institutions can support students through all stages of the student lifecycle.

This chapter examines the concept of transition and focuses on students' transitions into higher education. It argues that transitions are multiple, multidimensional and complex but, nevertheless, critical to the student experience. If students do not experience smooth transitions, this can result in mental ill-health. This chapter specifically focuses on the ways in which schools, colleges and universities can prepare students for their transition into higher education. The importance of induction and the first-year experience are also addressed.

WHAT IS TRANSITION?

It may seem surprising that there is no agreed definition of what constitutes a transition (Ecclestone et al, 2010). Colley (2007) conceptualises transition as simply 'a process of change over time' (p 428), while other researchers have defined transition as 'the capability to navigate change' (Gale and Parker, 2014, p 737). Transition has also been defined as 'a multidimensional process extending over a period' (Bonassi and Wolter, 2002, p 199).

4

While these perspectives emphasise the *process* of transition, traditional definitions have conceptualised transition as '*a fixed turning point which takes place at a preordained time and in a certain place*' (Quinn, 2010, p 122). However, the notion that transition takes place at a fixed point in time and at a fixed location has been rejected by transition theorists who conversely view transition as a *journey* (Furlong, 2009) along a pathway through several phases (Burnett, 2007).

The rejection of transition as a '*pivotal moment of change*' (Gale and Parker, 2014, p 739) has led to researchers giving increased attention to student transitions through the first year of higher education. It has been argued that the first year is '*arguably the most critical time*' (Krause, 2005, p 9) for students. It is a time when students experience multiple and multidimensional transitions. Many undergraduate students leave their home communities to study in a new town or city. They experience a physical transition. Additionally, they leave behind their social networks, which include peers, friendships and families. While technology enables them to stay socially connected with significant people, they will need to establish new social connections with people in student accommodation and peers who are studying the same course. Thus, they will need to navigate social transitions. Additionally, they will need to navigate academic transitions. Studying in higher education is fundamentally different in many ways to students' previous study. The curriculum content will be new, approaches to learning and teaching will place greater emphasis on students being independent learners and approaches to assessment are likely to be markedly different to what students have previously experienced.

Research has demonstrated how there is often a mismatch between student expectations and their initial experiences of higher education (Parkinson and Forrester, 2004) and this can result in student disengagement. Students may experience psychological transitions. For many students, moving away to university provides them with an opportunity to fashion their own identities and to develop their independence. Some students will need to adjust to the demands of independent living and personal budgeting for the first time. Motivation, confidence and self-esteem can be affected positively or negatively depending on how effectively students adapt to the changes that they are experiencing. If they have a positive experience of their course and institution and are able to quickly establish social connections, it is likely that students' experiences of transition will be positive. If their experiences in relation to these factors are negative, this can detrimentally impact on these psychological attributes.

SUPPORTING SMOOTH TRANSITIONS PRIOR TO ENTERING HIGHER EDUCATION

In adopting processes to support transition and develop learners' identities, schools, colleges and universities play a key role in equipping students with the skills and strategies to overcome or address transitional challenges (Briggs et al, 2012). After years of didactic teaching in primary and secondary classrooms (Kember, 2001; Harley et al, 2007), the importance of self-direction and independence within higher education can leave students feeling disorientated (Winn, 2002). Crucially, therefore, developing students' independence throughout their schooling is a priority if a smooth transition is to be experienced through and between these phases of education.

Through supporting universities' collaborative outreach programmes, open days, experience and taster sessions and pre-course events, schools and colleges play a vital role in developing students' independence through promoting an awareness of the routes through and between secondary, further and higher education courses.

COLLABORATIVE OUTREACH PROGRAMMES

Collaborative outreach programmes typically involve university representatives visiting schools and colleges to deliver informative and engaging guidance through activities and workshops. This can raise students' aspirations and encourage progression to higher education. Through supporting students' understanding of careers and pathways, outreach programmes develop students' confidence by addressing and exploring the questions and concerns that are often a source of anxiety for students.

OPEN DAYS, EXPERIENCE AND TASTER SESSIONS AND PRE-COURSE EVENTS

Many universities now organise open days, experience and taster sessions and pre-course events for students who plan to apply for or have firmly accepted offers of places.

Open days allow students to visit and experience universities first-hand to compare course and university provision. By providing students with academic advice and supporting accommodation and finance decisions, these events allow students considering higher education to develop their understanding of the higher education experience above and beyond the provisions of a prospectus. These events can also provide opportunities for parents and guardians to tour facilities and support students' aspirations through family engagement.

Following on from open days, experience and taster sessions usually take place on university campuses and allow students to engage with course-specific activities to introduce the expectations of higher education study. Often varying in length, these sessions can take place during term-time or throughout the summer and can provide students with an opportunity to live on campus and experience faculty and course facilities in a low-risk environment. By enabling students to explore the higher education experience, these sessions can develop students' aspirations and independence prior to submitting course and university applications.

Programme-specific, pre-course events take place following the acceptance of a course offer. These offer students opportunities to tour faculty buildings, meet programme staff and explore subject learning environments prior to commencing study as a higher education student. Crucially, they also allow students to network with peers within their subject and faculty area ahead of enrolment. Developing familiarity, and reducing exposure to the unknown, students build confidence and independence before embarking on their higher education study programme.

Encouraging students to engage with these events reduces barriers to participation in higher education, as confusion and anxiety often prevent or discourage students from engaging with such opportunities. This is particularly important for students who may be the first in their family to attend university. These students may lack cultural capital, particularly if they live in 'cold spot' areas where take-up of higher education is low. Their families may not be able to adequately support them with the process of applying for and transitioning to life at university. Consequently, these students may lack the networks of support from their families that other students may take for granted. For students who are first in their family to attend higher education, schools and colleges play a critical role in empowering these students so that they believe they can benefit from higher education. Considering the challenges facing first-generation students, including the potential of parents, guardians and carers to influence or limit study (Mitchall and Jaeger, 2018), efforts by schools, colleges and universities to engage these stakeholders and develop cultural capital are a priority.

7

SOCIAL NETWORKING

Some courses, faculties and universities encourage new students to join closed social network groups during the summer period prior to starting a course in the autumn term. This provides a valuable opportunity for students to develop social connections and discuss common anxieties in a safe environment. The use of social media to support peer networking allows students to connect and communicate within a context with which they are already familiar.

CRITICAL QUESTIONS

+ How can higher education institutions support schools and colleges in developing students' independence to prepare them for higher education?

+ In what ways can higher education institutions support schools and colleges to encourage first-generation applicants to apply for entry to higher education?

+ How might higher education institutions support schools and colleges to promote student engagement with social media groups prior to them entering higher education?

Approximately three-quarters of adults with mental ill-health experience symptoms before the age of 25.

Mental health conditions account for an increasing proportion of all disability disclosed by first-year students (17 per cent in 2015/16, compared to 5 per cent in 2006/07).

Female first-year students are more likely than male first-year students to disclose a mental health condition (2.5 per cent compared to 1.4 per cent in 2015/16).

Just under half of students who report experiencing a mental health condition choose not to disclose it to their university.

94 per cent of universities report an increase in demand for counselling services, with 61 per cent reporting an increase in demand of over 25 per cent. In some universities, up to one in four students are using, or waiting to use, counselling services

(www.ippr.org/files/2017-09/not-by-degrees-summary-sept-2017-1-.pdf)

CRITICAL QUESTIONS

+ What facts might make male students more reluctant to disclose a mental illness?

+ Why might students be reluctant to declare to their university that they have a mental illness?

+ How might universities increase declaration rates?

Research has demonstrated that the first year of higher education can often be a difficult and complex period for students from diverse social backgrounds (Kift, 2009; Kift and Nelson, 2005). Finnegan and Merrill (2015) describe transitions for working-class students to university as risky. Research by Meehan and Howells (2018) found that students from widening participation backgrounds, who are more likely to commute to university rather than live in university accommodation, are more likely to have a negative educational experience than students who live in student accommodation. Some students from working-class backgrounds experience university as an *alien* environment (Askham, 2008), particularly where they perceive it to be a largely middle-class environment.

(Reay et al, 2005)

CRITICAL QUESTIONS

+ What factors might result in a negative experience of university for students from different social and cultural backgrounds?

+ What can universities do to promote a sense of belonging for students from widening participation backgrounds?

CASE STUDY

A university developed a residential summer school in July for students who were starting their degree programmes in September. Students who held conditional and unconditional offers of places were invited to attend a one-week pre-course induction programme. The programme was carefully designed and included a range of activities to facilitate both academic and social development. Students were introduced to

9

lecture theatres through a programme of keynote lectures. The academic skills team provided sessions on the importance of learning outcomes, how to search for literature, essay writing and academic referencing. The student union provided a range of activities to develop social skills and confidence. The students stayed in the university accommodation so that they could develop social connections prior to starting their course.

CRITICAL QUESTIONS

+ How might students' expectations of support align with tutors' expectations of independence?

+ How can universities provide students with realistic expectations?

+ How can universities help students develop their cultural capital and overcome the 'first-generation' challenge?

THE ROLE OF INDUCTION IN SUPPORTING A SMOOTH TRANSITION

It has been argued that induction should be a process rather than a one-off event (Leese, 2010). Induction activities typically focus on a variety of tasks including:

+ library induction;

+ student support services including disability support;

+ counselling and academic support;

+ student union activities;

+ specific activities related to course induction.

Typically, students on undergraduate courses in the UK experience an induction week or 'freshers' week at the beginning of their studies. They filter out information that they do not perceive as relevant and they often experience information saturation during the early stages of their studies. The advantage of spreading induction throughout the duration of the first year is that students can be provided with the information they need as and when it is required.

The induction process should help students to assimilate into university life. Induction programmes therefore need to be flexible to respond to the needs of different students, including adult learners who are studying at university alongside managing family commitments, commuter students and those living away from home. Students come to university with different interests, values and beliefs. Thus, it is essential to provide them with a menu of taster activities that cater for the diverse range of student needs.

Developing a sense of belonging is critical to inclusion and students who feel that they belong to the institution are more likely to complete their studies. The aim of an induction programme should be to engender a sense of belonging so that students feel that they are suited to their new environment. It is critical that induction sessions are positive and encouraging so that students do not feel intimidated from the start. The way that all staff interact with them during these early stages of their university life is crucial and therefore interactions should be consistently positive and supportive.

ACADEMIC INDUCTION

Students need to be supported to understand how their learning at university will be different to previous study at school and college. Over time, they will increasingly be expected to self-direct their own learning. They will undertake a variety of assessments in different modes and they might be expected to undertake periods of assessed work experience. They should not expect their lecturers to 'spoon-feed' them all the relevant academic content and they should gradually expect to take greater ownership of their assessment tasks. They will need to understand their responsibilities in preparing for lectures, seminars and tutorials and their responsibilities in relation to time management. They will need to learn how to manage their own study time and their own attendance. Induction programmes that are carefully designed can address many of these areas.

Academic writing is particularly challenging, and many students arrive at university without the skills of information searching, critical analysis and academic referencing. Most first-year programmes cover these aspects during induction and students may be required to study a module that addresses these aspects as part of their first-year course. However, it is important not to overload students with too much information during the initial induction week as this can be daunting. Students can be 'drip-fed' with information, so that they gain the knowledge they require at the time they need to use it.

Kift (2009) emphasises the importance of a cumulative approach to transition which incorporates the gradual withdrawal of scaffolding. This needs to be explicitly stated during the induction process so that institutions can manage students' expectations. Lecturers should also be explicit about when and how they can be contacted, when students can expect to receive replies and how much support students can expect from them at different stages of their academic programme. Managing expectations in this way means that students do not develop unrealistic expectations at the start.

Course induction should map out the terrain for students. They need to understand the programme learning outcomes and the journey they will travel throughout their course. Providing them with a 'road map' is helpful so that they begin to understand what knowledge and skills they will develop throughout their course. It is useful to provide students with an overview of all the modules they will study and the assessment tasks that they will undertake at the start of their studies. Students need to also understand how the different modules they study relate to each other and how the modules contribute to programme learning outcomes.

THE ROLE OF TUTORS AND SUPPORT STAFF

With the experiences of many first-year students being neither satis-fying nor successful (Kantanis, 2000), strategies to support transition prior to entering higher education must develop and remain a priority throughout students' first-year studies.

To combat anxiety, uncertainty and disengagement (Meehan and Howells, 2018), tutor approachability and academic guidance is pivotal if transition is to be successful throughout first-year study. Tutors and support staff therefore play a crucial role in supporting the develop-ment of students' study skills through providing guidance on the time-management and organisational skills that may not have underpinned previous study.

Through supporting engagement and independence, personal tutors can equip students with the knowledge they need to understand the value of assessment and feedback. Personal tutors can support students to develop resilience to feedback so that they can act upon and learn from academic feedback. Students may need support from tutors to help them to understand the differences between education in schools and colleges and education in universities, where there are greater expectations on students to be self-motivated and independent. Drawing upon these experiences and differences, students can begin to understand their own role in the learning process and the interrelationship between this and their own success.

Universities continue to prioritise the provision of student support services and these provide students with access to many confidential and personalised services covering a range of both academic and personal issues. Universities often offer counselling and medical services, study support services, disability support, advice for students with dyslexia and specific learning difficulties, and guidance on administration, finance and accommodation. These one-stop student shops can allow students to access information and support on many issues, including those that are likely to be new experiences.

The importance of students establishing friendships during the first year is critical to them being mentally healthy. Students can experience a sense of isolation if they do not establish friendships and this does not only apply to those who choose to live away from home. Opportunities to develop social connectivity can be embedded into course design and it is therefore crucial that students are given opportunities to work collaboratively in classes and on assessment tasks during the first year. Group projects and group assessments can be effective tools for developing social connections. Taking students off-site on educational visits can be particularly effective and residential programmes can help to foster teamwork skills.

- The number of students withdrawing from university courses with mental health problems has more than trebled in recent years.

- Over the past ten years there has been a fivefold increase in the proportion of students who disclose a mental health condition to their institution.

- In 2017/18, 49,265 undergraduate and 8,040 postgraduate students disclosed that they were experiencing mental ill-health.

- In recent years, there has been a steady increase in the number of student suicides. Some universities in the UK have experienced several student suicides within a short period of time.

(www.universitiesuk.ac.uk/policy-and-analysis/reports/Documents/2018/ minding-our-future-starting-conversation-student-mental-health.pdf)

CRITICAL QUESTIONS

+ What factors do you think might account for the increase in student mental ill-health?

+ What factors might result specifically in postgraduate students developing mental ill-health?

+ How might universities support students to positively manage their own mental health?

It has been claimed that social integration and academic performance are strong predictors of student attrition (Hillman, 2005). Thus, both are required to support successful transition into university life. Induction programmes should therefore focus on the curriculum, pedagogy, assessment and co-curricular activities that enable students to establish social connections through engaging in purposeful activities.

CASE STUDY

A university introduced subject peer learning mentors. The mentors had to apply for the position and they received financial reimbursement for the hours they worked. The peer mentors were final-year students. They mentored students in the first and second years who were also studying the same course. They provided timetabled 'drop-in' sessions to students who required additional support. They also offered email and video conferencing support during specific timetabled slots. Feedback from students indicated that they enjoyed receiving support from their peers and they enjoyed the fact that they could develop a more informal relationship with their mentors compared to the more formal relationship they developed with their tutors.

SUMMARY

This chapter has emphasised the importance of facilitating smooth transitions into higher education. Smooth transitions at all stages of the student lifecycle help to reduce the prevalence of mental health difficulties in students. It has argued that the induction process should extend throughout the first-year experience rather than being a single event at the start of the course. It has highlighted the important role that open days, outreach activities and pre-course events can play in supporting students to feel confident and positive about higher education.

CHECKLIST

This chapter has addressed:

✓ the significance of pre-course events in supporting student transitions into higher education;

✓ the importance of establishing positive partnerships between schools, colleges and universities to provide students with a rich menu of pre-course events;

✓ the necessity to extend the process of induction throughout the first-year experience.

FURTHER READING

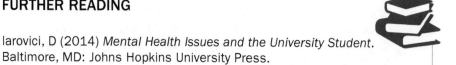

Iarovici, D (2014) *Mental Health Issues and the University Student*. Baltimore, MD: Johns Hopkins University Press.

+ CHAPTER 2

RISK FACTORS

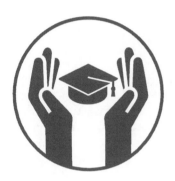

PROFESSIONAL LINKS

This chapter addresses the following:

Universities UK (2015) *Student Mental Wellbeing in Higher Education: Good Practice Guide*.

CHAPTER OBJECTIVES

After reading this chapter you will understand:

+ the risk factors that might contribute to mental ill-health in students;

+ what lecturers can do to address these risk factors.

INTRODUCTION

This chapter addresses the risk factors that might result in mental ill-health in students. Some of these risk factors are individual to the student, some are institutional, while others are related to students' social and cultural backgrounds. This chapter provides guidance to higher education tutors so that they can minimise the risk of mental ill-health in students.

ASSESSMENT PRESSURES

Assessments are a critical aspect of the student experience. Successful completion of assessment tasks enables students to progress from one level of study to the next and the grades that students achieve in these tasks influence the overall classification of the award at the end of the period of study. While students may be used to taking terminal examinations in school, they are much more likely to experience modular assessment in higher education. Module assessments can cause students a considerable amount of stress. Modes of assessment may vary, depending on the course being studied, and typically include examinations, essays, presentations, placements and other types of coursework. While some courses may include final examinations, it is likely that module assessments completed during their studies also contribute to students' overall grade. Module assessments can be particularly challenging for students if there is a 'bunching' of assessment tasks. Course leaders should aim to spread out deadlines to alleviate unnecessary stress being placed on students.

Modular assessment tasks are designed to address module learning outcomes which underpin programme or course learning outcomes. Course leaders should ensure that assessment tasks reflect a range of modes of assessment so that students are not continually expected to demonstrate a narrow range of academic skills. For example, essays are over-used as a mode of assessment in higher education. This means that students who do not perform well in essays are not given enough opportunities to thrive. While academic writing is an important feature of most degree courses, inclusive assessment uses a range of modes of assessment across a course so that all students can achieve their potential. Using a variety of modes of assessment also keeps students engaged and enables them to develop a wider range of skills.

If you are a course leader you should ensure that assessment tasks are carefully designed for students' knowledge, skills and understanding across a course.

ASSESSMENT CRITERIA

If you are a module leader or module tutor, providing students with clear assessment criteria helps them to understand exactly what they are expected to do to demonstrate achievement at a specific level. The problem with assessment criteria is that they are often phrased using academic jargon, resulting in students being unclear of the expectations of a specific assessment task. This can develop students' anxieties and contribute to feelings of stress. Providing vague criteria can also worsen these feelings and contribute to students' mental ill-health.

CRITICAL QUESTIONS

Consider the following assessment criteria:

  80–100 per cent: a polished and excellent understanding of the subject content;

  70–79 per cent: a very good understanding of the subject content;

  60–69 per cent: a good understanding of the subject;

  50–59 per cent: a sound understanding of the subject content;

  40–49 per cent: a limited understanding of the subject content.

+ What are the problems with these assessment criteria?

+ How might you improve these criteria so that students are clear about what they need to do?

CRITERION- AND NORM-REFERENCED ASSESSMENT

These criteria are known as criterion-referenced assessment criteria. Essentially, this means that the work is graded and if the work meets the criteria at a specific level, this is the grade that is awarded. This is different to norm-referenced assessment where work is marked for a cohort and then marks are then adjusted to create a normal distribution of marks in the form of a bell curve.

CRITICAL QUESTIONS

+ What are the advantages and disadvantages of criterion-referenced assessment?

+ What are the advantages and disadvantages of norm-referenced assessment?

CONTEXTUALISING ASSESSMENT CRITERIA

Some assessment criteria might include phrases such as 'excellent critical analysis' or 'good critical analysis'. The problem with these phrases is that students often do not know what 'excellent' or 'good' means in the context of the specific assessment task they are undertaking. Students often do not understand what 'critical analysis' looks like in a specific assessment task. This can result in students experiencing stress and anxiety. One solution to this problem is to contextualise the assessment criteria to a specific assessment task.

Below is an example of contextualised criteria for an education essay on autism.

70–79 per cent:

Knowledge	Understands the three main barriers to learning. Identifies evidence-based strategies to address these.
Use of literature	Includes a wide range of sources from peer-reviewed journals, books and government reports.
Critical analysis	Includes detailed critical analysis of at least three research studies which are explored in depth. Demonstrates a critical understanding about the use of labelling.
Application of theory	Applies Theory of Mind to classroom practice.

CRITICAL QUESTIONS

+ What are the advantages of contextualising assessment criteria in this way?

+ How might you differentiate these criteria at different levels?

TRANSITIONS TO HIGHER EDUCATION ASSESSMENT

Supporting students' understanding of the assessment methods used in higher education is crucial in promoting positive mental health. Through experiencing uncertainty and lacking confidence, students often require support if they are to successfully approach assessment within higher education. These feelings may be exacerbated for students in their first year of study.

As a tutor, providing writing frames or structure guides can significantly reduce students' anxieties while also developing awareness of subject and tutor demands. Through liaison with other academic staff, the use of these frames and guides can be gradually withdrawn as students progress through higher education. While using guides and frames supports students' transition both into and through their university study, a planned and purposeful phased withdrawal can ensure students are still given essential opportunities to develop their independence.

GROUP ASSESSMENT

Increasingly, universities are using group assessment in response to the challenge of increasing class sizes. While these allow universities to vary their approaches to assessment, group assessments also provide an opportunity for students to develop time management, organisation and communication skills. Despite these benefits, group assessments can present staff with difficulties in determining whether and how to assess students and allocate marks to individual students. Often sharing these same concerns, students' anxieties can be worsened through feelings of dependence on the engagement and participation of their peers despite having no control over these.

As a tutor, you can alleviate these anxieties and support students' positive mental health. Clear guidance must be established and disseminated detailing how individual students will be assessed and awarded marks in instances where there may be concerns about the contribution made by other group members. By ensuring that there is a clear process in place for any student who may wish to share these concerns, student confidence can be supported through removing barriers to successful group assessment.

EXEMPLAR MATERIALS

In supporting students' academic writing, exemplar assessment materials can be provided by tutors to provide students with material against which they can create, pitch and structure their own work. This can support students in overcoming a range of barriers to the successful completion of assessments by alleviating anxieties and promoting positive mental health, and is particularly valuable to those facing a range of assessment modes for the first time. Again, developing students' independence remains a crucial focus and a phased withdrawal of these materials may be appropriate.

ORAL BRIEFINGS

Tutors can use oral briefings to deconstruct assessment criteria. Oral briefings can develop students' familiarity with higher education assessment and ensure that students are able to approach assessments with confidence. These briefings allow students to explore and compare their ideas with peers, as well as develop their knowledge and understanding of their tutor's expectations. Deconstructing assessment criteria in this way also provides students with an opportunity to discuss their concerns with peers and tutors to ensure that success criteria have been understood prior to students drafting and writing assessed work.

VIDEO PODCASTS

As a tutor, you can make use of video recording software to share video podcasts with students. The use of video podcasts ensures that the tutor's advice and guidance remains accessible throughout key periods of assessment. By providing accessible advice and guidance using video podcasts, students' confidence and independence can be developed, which alleviates anxieties and supports positive mental health.

LEARNING OUTCOMES

Providing clear, transparent and precise learning outcomes allows students to value and understand the relationship between their studies and any assessment activities. This provides students with an opportunity to monitor and understand how their success will be measured following their studies. Student involvement here is critical if students are to approach assessments equipped with an understanding of how to meet learning outcomes. Tutors should take steps to ensure learning outcomes are accessible and can be understood by students, and opportunities for dialogue can be useful to allow students to ask questions. This is particularly important in instances where students may be new to the assessment mode being used.

FEEDBACK AND FEEDFORWARD

Feedback and feedforward processes are often used to provide students with personalised guidance and areas of development. However, students often lack the skills required to address this guidance and maximise academic success. Tutors therefore play a crucial role in ensuring that students are aware of how to respond to and action any guidance provided. Some focus on developing students' skills may be needed before students can benefit fully from tutor guidance. Through ensuring that feedback and feedforward activities maintain focus on students' efforts and strengths, tutors also play a vital role in developing students' self-belief, which supports engagement and positive mental health.

Tutors should seek to offer personalised feedback, including the use of students' names, to create a culture of recognition and ownership in which students' ideas and contributions are valued. In doing so, tutors should ensure any feedback seeks to justify grades awarded to maintain transparency and support students' understanding of their own strengths and areas of development.

By providing students with targets that are designed to support improvement, tutors should also consider providing examples and exemplar material to ensure that students understand their targets and are able to apply these within the context of their own studies. Tutors can also ensure that feedback is accessible to students through using student-friendly language and avoiding jargon.

CASE STUDY

A group of undergraduate sociology students were experiencing stress due to a high volume of coursework. They complained that the assessment tasks in all modules were due in at the same time at the end of the semester. This meant that they had no assessment tasks during the semester but at the end of the semester they had multiple deadlines to meet. The course leader decided to spread the assessment load by introducing patchwork assessments in two of the modules for this group of students. Rather than submitting one large assessment task in a module, the students were set a series of smaller tasks that they were required to submit once every two weeks. In one of these modules these tasks included a video podcast, a blog, a piece of short critical writing and a poster presentation. At the end of the module these tasks were collated and submitted in the form of an electronic portfolio. The students were required to write an over-arching narrative to 'stitch' the separate tasks together. The students enjoyed working on these varied tasks, and student engagement and attendance also improved. The different modes of assessment reflected a 'patchwork' of tasks. In the over-arching narrative, the students were required to reflect on their own development in relation to the module learning outcomes.

COURSE FACTORS

Course-related factors can create mental ill-health in students. As a course leader you will need to be aware of these and take steps to alleviate them. It will not be possible to eradicate stress from students' lives and not all stress is bad stress. A degree of stress can be healthy because it challenges the students to achieve things that they might not have considered were possible. However, mental ill-health is when stress, anxiety and depression prevent students from participating in their usual daily activities. You should have processes in place for consulting with students and collecting their feedback during the year. This feedback is usually collected through surveys or focus groups with students. It is worth considering including a question on course-related factors that affect their well-being so that you can identify any issues that need addressing. You will need to ascertain from students what the factors are and what their suggestions are for alleviating student mental ill-health.

Strategies that help to maintain positive student mental health include:

+ spreading out assessment deadlines;

+ developing clear mechanisms for regularly communicating course-related news to students;

+ following up on non-attendance and ascertaining if the student needs further support;

+ meeting with students who do not submit coursework on time to ascertain if they need further support;

+ meeting with students who have a declining academic profile.

If you are a module tutor you should monitor student engagement in lectures and seminars and in cases where engagement is low a conversation with the student can help to ascertain if there are any problems that you need to be aware of.

All conversations should be non-judgemental and non-threatening. The purpose of talking to students is to find out if the student needs any additional mental health support to increase their participation and outcomes.

CAMPUS CLIMATE

In universities where the campus climate is positive, students experience a sense of belonging. This sense of belonging is critical for good mental health and for student retention. Students who do not experience a sense of belonging are more likely to withdraw from their course. They are also more likely to under-achieve. To achieve a positive campus climate, you should consider the following:

+ treating all students with respect;

+ recognising all students as stakeholders;

+ empowering all students by giving them a voice;

+ the extent to which courses reflect student diversity;

+ embedding images of student diversity when designing prospectuses, web pages, course and module handbooks and student digital videos used for marketing;

+ ensuring that visual displays around campus reflect a diverse student body;

+ representing students from minority groups on university and student committees;

+ communicating the institutional commitment to equality on signs, notices and posters around the campus and including messages about zero tolerance of prejudice-based bullying, harassment and discrimination;

+ demonstrating an institutional commitment to religious and cultural festivals.

INDIVIDUAL FACTORS

Students with disabilities are particularly vulnerable to developing mental ill-health and may require a personalised learning and support plan to enable them to succeed. Students with autism may require support to navigate the social environment of the university campus and you may need to adapt approaches to learning, teaching and assessment tasks to reduce the distress that they may experience from tasks that require social interaction with peers. These students may also need a staged transition to university to prevent them from developing mental ill-health. Chapter 5 addresses this in more depth.

Some students may need to access additional academic and pastoral support to enable them to succeed at university. As a tutor you will teach students with a range of needs including those with dyslexia, physical or sensory impairments, or social, emotional and mental health needs. You may be responsible for teaching students with specific communication and language needs. If these students have been assessed by disability services, they may have a personal learning and support plan. If you are a course leader you must share these plans with relevant teaching staff. If you are a module tutor, you will need to address the recommendations of the plan by adapting teaching and assessment. If you are a personal tutor, you are responsible for checking with the student that the recommendations are being addressed and if they are not you will need to follow up on this with relevant colleagues. You might also need to make referrals to other services in the university. Talking to the student to find out what adaptations they think they need is also a very effective way of empowering the student.

FAMILY AND COMMUNITY FACTORS

Student mental health is also influenced by family and community factors. Family and community factors that affect mental health might include:

+ family conflict;

+ social deprivation;

+ abuse and neglect;

+ caring responsibilities to parents, siblings or children;

+ being separated from family members;

+ homesickness;

+ unrealistic expectations from family members;

+ relationship breakdown in student accommodation;

+ crime in the community.

This is not an exhaustive list and it is also important to remember that mental ill-health occurs across the full spectrum of social backgrounds. If you are a personal tutor and a student presents with mental ill-health, you need to ascertain the reasons for this by exploring whether the students' needs are a result of course, individual, family or community factors. Once you know the cause, you can then start a conversation with the student about possible solutions. However, it is important to remember that personal tutors are not counsellors. If the student is demonstrating severe and prolonged mental ill-health that is detrimentally impacting on their participation in various aspects of life, then you will need to refer the student (with their consent) to specialist mental health support services.

CRITICAL QUESTIONS

+ Can you give three examples of student cases that you would refer to the mental health services in the university?

+ Why might students be reluctant to access mental health services in the university?

- 90.5 per cent of students believe university exams and assessments are 'reasonably' or 'very' stressful.
- 30 per cent of students interviewed felt that issues including exams and assessment had a negative impact on their life.

(www.nus.org.uk/PageFiles/12238/THINK-POS-REPORT-Final.pdf)

CRITICAL QUESTIONS

+ How can universities improve communication between departments and faculties to prevent overlaps during key assessment periods?

+ How can universities refine their approaches to assessment to improve students' positive mental health?

Margaret Price has argued that tutors need to develop students' assessment literacy skills not only so that they understand the requirements of their assessment tasks but also so that they are clear on what they need to do to achieve a specific grade band (Price et al, 2012). Activities to develop assessment literacy skills include helping students to understand and use assessment criteria through tasks such as self- and peer-assessment and analysis of exemplar assessments. These practices take the mystery out of assessment and therefore reduce student anxieties.

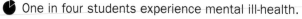
- One in four students experience mental ill-health.
- 34 per cent of female students compared to 19 per cent of males experience mental ill-health.
- LGBTQ+ students are twice as likely to experience mental ill-health compared to heterosexual students.

(https://yougov.co.uk/topics/lifestyle/articles-reports/2016/08/09/
quarter-britains-students-are-afflicted-mental-hea)

Erin Potts (2017) has argued that colleges and universities have a responsibility to provide a campus climate which welcomes and supports a student's disclosure of mental ill-health. The onset of mental health problems often occurs during a student's undergraduate studies, and prevalence among students aged between 15 and 24 is notably high. Having experienced an increase in the number of students with mental ill-health, many universities now provide on-campus mental health support services for students. Students often face a difficult decision in deciding whether to disclose a mental health problem. Potts argues that universities have a duty to deconstruct mental health stigmas and provide environments within which students feel comfortable making declarations and seeking support.

CASE STUDY

One university which offers joint honours degrees and interdisciplinary degrees across and through two partner institutions has developed a process to support communication between its separate schools, faculties, campuses and institutions. With students often completing modules and units across different departments, with each determining its own assessment schedules, students often found that deadlines and exam dates either overlapped or fell on the same day or within the same week. Responding to student satisfaction feedback, the university has created opportunities for a representative from each area to meet twice a year to discuss and jointly agree assessment timetables. This ensures students are not placed under excess pressure through the unnecessary overlapping of assessment deadlines. This allows students to submit assessed work throughout each academic year, which significantly reduces students' anxieties and improves well-being.

SUMMARY

This chapter has outlined some of the risk factors that can result in mental ill-health in students. You have learned about institutional, individual, family and community factors that can have a detrimental impact on students' mental health. Course leaders, module tutors and personal tutors can provide non-therapeutic support which can alleviate mental ill-health. If students are demonstrating prolonged and severe mental ill-health that is affecting their participation in daily life and might be putting them at risk, cases should be referred, with student consent, to specialist mental health support services in the university.

CHECKLIST

This chapter has addressed:

✓ ways of reducing stress in relation to assessment and feedback;

✓ institutional, individual, family, community and course-related risk factors that can result in mental ill-health;

✓ the role of course leaders, module tutors and personal tutors in alleviating mental ill-health in students.

FURTHER READING

Poole, R (2013) *Mental Health and Poverty*. Cambridge: Cambridge University Press.

✚ CHAPTER 3

COMMON MENTAL HEALTH NEEDS IN STUDENTS

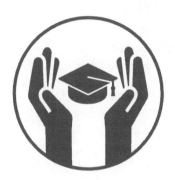

PROFESSIONAL LINKS

This chapter addresses the following:

HM Government (2011) *No Health without Mental Health: A Cross-Government Mental Health Outcomes Strategy for People of All Ages*. Department of Health.

CHAPTER OBJECTIVES

After reading this chapter you will understand:

+ common mental health needs experienced by students;

+ how to identify these needs;

+ how to support students with mental ill-health.

INTRODUCTION

In this chapter you will learn about the causes of mental ill-health in the student population and the common types of mental illness that students experience. You will learn about some of the warning signs to support you in identifying needs early. You will also learn about how you can support students with mental health needs.

It is deeply concerning that mental illness appears to be increasing in the student population. While the causes of student mental illness are well documented, the reasons for this apparent increase are less clear and there is a need to research this further. Mental illness can detrimentally impact on student well-being, attainment and overall life chances. Through identifying needs early, students can be supported to get the help they need before the problem escalates.

Going to university can be stressful for all students. It is important not to overlook the needs of postgraduate students, part-time students and students who are studying courses by distance learning. Students on these courses can experience feelings of isolation, particularly if their interactions with lecturers and peers are less frequent. Any student or staff member can develop mental ill-health. With the right support these students can complete their studies successfully and achieve good academic and employment outcomes. This chapter outlines the causes of mental ill-health in students and addresses common mental health needs.

WHAT IS MENTAL HEALTH?

The World Health Organization (WHO) provides a positive definition of mental health:

Mental health is defined as a state of well-being in which every individual realizes his or her own potential, can cope with the normal stresses of life, can work productively and fruitfully, and is able to make a contribution to her or his community... Health is a state of complete physical, mental and social well-being and not merely the absence of disease or infirmity.

(WHO, 2014)

While some definitions of mental health emphasise mental *illness*, the WHO definition focuses on well-being for all. It extends the concept of mental health to everyone rather than associating the term only with people who demonstrate signs of mental illness. Chapter 4 specifically examines the institution-wide approach to mental health which, through its implementation, ensures that all individuals within an organisation can stay mentally healthy. This chapter focuses on mental illness.

CAUSES OF MENTAL ILL-HEALTH

The causes of mental ill-health in students are multifaceted. Moving away from home for the first time can be stressful for students and can result in isolation. This can lead to depression until new social networks are formed. Many students who go to university will be responsible for self-management for the first time. They may have to cope with domestic tasks and financial management, and developing these skills can be challenging for some students. University may also be a time when students are starting to explore their sexual and gender identities. They may be starting sexual relationships for the first time and they may have to cope with relationship break-ups or conflict within relationships. At the same time they are required to adapt to new ways of teaching, independent study and new approaches to assessment. Learning how to navigate all these changes can be stressful and it can result in anxiety and depression. Some students may experience depression because they are living significant distances away from their families or friendship groups that they established prior to going to university. They may experience homesickness and it may take them a while to adapt to their new geographical location. Some students may be dissatisfied with their choice of course and this can result in significant anxiety. Some may be balancing academic study alongside caring responsibilities to children or other family members. All these factors can result in mental ill-health.

DECLARING MENTAL HEALTH NEEDS

Students may be reluctant to disclose that they have a mental illness because they are worried that this will affect the way others view them, particularly their lecturers. It is important that the institution promotes positive messages about mental health so that any stigma associated with mental health is eradicated. Higher education providers are not legally able to discriminate either directly or indirectly against students based on mental health and the institution has a duty of care to all of its students. Under the Equality Act (2010), all educational institutions are legally obligated to make reasonable adjustments to provide equality of opportunity for students with disabilities. Students need to understand these legal responsibilities so that they do not become anxious about the perceived consequences of making a disclosure.

Universities cannot make students disclose a mental illness. The decision about whether to disclose information about their mental health can only be made by the student. However, universities should help students to understand that disclosure will enable the university to provide more effective, bespoke support so that they are able to thrive. Positive messages about mental health can be transmitted to students during open days, on the university website, through social media and in the university prospectus.

CRITICAL QUESTIONS

+ Why might some students studying on professional courses (such as nursing, teaching and social work) be reluctant to disclose a mental illness to university staff?

+ Why might students studying on these courses be reluctant to disclose a mental illness to a placement provider?

+ What are the legal responsibilities of universities and placement providers in relation to student mental health?

DEPRESSION

Depression is not the same thing as low mood. Most people experience a low mood from time to time in response to experiences in their lives.

Depression occurs when low mood is prolonged and starts to affect an individual's participation in day-to-day life. Some common symptoms of depression are listed in Table 3.1.

TABLE 3.1 Some common symptoms of depression

Emotional	Cognitive	Physiological	Behavioural
Depressed mood	Reduced concentration	Low energy/ fatigue	Social withdrawal
Persistent sad, anxious or empty mood	Difficulty making decisions	Restlessness	Non-participation in activities (including poor attendance)
Sudden changes in mood	Poor self-concept and self-esteem	Insomnia	
	Poor self-confidence	Hypersomnia	
Tearfulness	Feeling of hope-lessness or helplessness	Poor appetite	Decline in self-care or personal appearance
	Feeling loss of control	Over-eating	
	Feelings of guilt and pessimism		Demotivation
	Suicidal thoughts		

Some students with depression find it difficult to concentrate during learning activities and they may isolate themselves from their peers. They tend to question their own ability and may lack motivation in classes and in relation to assessment tasks. They may attend classes infrequently and fail to submit assessments on time. Their academic performance may demonstrate a decline over time.

If you suspect that a student is experiencing depression you should try to talk to them individually. This might be difficult (and frustrating) because they may have stopped responding to emails and they may refuse to answer the phone. However, you need to be persistent. When you meet with the student, consider using the following example to structure the conversation:

1. *Hello Sam, it is good to see you today.*
2. *I have been worried about you. I have noticed that you [seem unhappy etc].* Avoid highlighting negatives such as lack of attendance or declining grades.
3. *Is there anything we need to know about to help us understand a little more what is happening?*
4. Listen to the student and allow them to talk.
5. *How do you think we can support you more effectively on the course? What can we do to help?*
6. *What would you like us to do next? What would you like to do next?*

If a student is demonstrating signs of chronic depression, a referral to student services might be an appropriate course of action if the student has consented to this. You should be willing to be flexible with deadlines, punctuality and student attendance until the issue is resolved. If the student is unable to attend classes, you should ensure that they are provided with lecture content on the virtual learning platform, including videos, podcasts and lecture slides so that they can work from home. You should monitor them carefully by 'checking-in' with them at least once a week, either via phone, video conferencing or email.

CRITICAL QUESTIONS

+ What strategies might you suggest to students to alleviate depression?
+ What factors might result in depression in students?

ANXIETY

It is normal for everyone to experience anxiety from time to time, particularly in response to stressful events. Some people experience general anxiety in which they are anxious in most situations. Others experience phobias only in relation to very specific experiences which trigger physiological, emotional, cognitive and behavioural responses. Some of the signs of anxiety are shown in Table 3.2.

TABLE 3.2 Some common symptoms of anxiety

Emotional	Cognitive	Physiological	Behavioural
Worry Nervousness	Concentration difficulties Memory problems Perfectionist traits	Rapid heart rate Rapid and shallow breathing Excess perspiration Muscle tension Headaches Stomach pain Sleep problems	Restlessness Irritability Task avoidance Fear of failure Withdrawal

Some people with anxiety over-estimate the level of danger and under-estimate their abilities to cope with specific situations. Physiological responses, such as excessive perspiration, can further increase the level of anxiety.

Different experiences might trigger anxiety in students. Examples include:

+ delivering a presentation to peers/public speaking;

+ fear of examinations;

+ fear of being observed by a mentor on a placement;

+ external factors at home, in the community or elsewhere;

+ fear of failure.

CRITICAL QUESTIONS

+ What other factors might trigger student anxiety?

+ To what extent can a degree of anxiety facilitate productivity?

If you notice that a student is anxious, you should try to speak to them privately to find out how they feel and to ask for their perspective on how you can help them. Many students experience anxiety during assessed presentations. You can alleviate some of the anxiety by giving them the option to present to a smaller group or to present using a recorded video file. Some students get particularly anxious about assessment tasks.

Providing very clear assignment guidance and exemplar assignments will help to alleviate the anxiety. Some students might be anxious about being placed in a particular class. It might be possible to move them to a different group to reduce this anxiety. Some students might experience anxiety simply stepping into a university, particularly if the campus is large. Universities can be daunting! You can support students by being a friendly face when they arrive on campus, taking them for a coffee or assigning them to a peer mentor who can meet with them when they are on campus. Students who are demonstrating chronic anxiety may need to be referred to student support services, particularly if the anxiety is so great that it is affecting their participation in aspects of university life.

SELF-HARM

There are many myths relating to self-harm which you need to be aware of. These are identified below.

+ Self-harm is not usually a manipulative act.

+ It is not usually a form of attention-seeking, as many young people try to hide the evidence of the self-harm

+ It is not usually a failed suicide attempt – people who self-harm are not usually suicidal.

+ It is not usually carried out for pleasure.

+ It is not an indication of a personality disorder.

+ The seriousness of the injury is not related to the seriousness of the problem.

+ It is not carried out because victims like pain; it is often a way of coping.

+ Self-harm is not a young person's issue; people of all ages self-harm.

+ It is not easy to stop self-harming.

+ The problems do not go away if the self-harm stops.

The reasons for self-harm vary across individuals but a common reason is to turn an emotional pain into a physical pain. This can help to distract individuals from the emotional pain they are experiencing. Students might also use self-harm as a form of punishment (www.mind.org.uk). It can be difficult to identify self-harm, as some people will go to significant lengths to cover up the evidence.

Warning signs may include:

+ unexplained burns, cuts, scars, or other clusters of similar markings on the skin;

+ arms, hands and forearms opposite the dominant hand are common areas for self-harm, although self-harm can take place on other parts of the body;

+ inappropriate dress for the season, such as consistently wearing long sleeves or trousers in the summer;

+ constant use of wristbands or other coverings;

+ unwillingness to participate in events or activities that require less clothing;

+ frequently wearing bandages;

+ increased signs of depression or anxiety.

It is important to be non-judgemental if you identify self-harm or if a student discloses it to you. If they make a disclosure do not tell them to *just stop doing it*: they are doing it as a coping mechanism, not as a form of manipulating other people. It is not easy for them to stop doing it. The underlying causes need to be addressed first. Make a plan: involve the student in developing a plan of 'ways forward'. Depending on the severity of the self-harm, the student may need to be referred to student services. If a student is actively suicidal, stay calm and make sure they are safe and with someone so that you can go and seek advice. In some cases, a student may have already overdosed and in such cases an ambulance will be needed.

EATING DISORDERS

Eating disorders are complex and the reasons for developing them vary across individuals. They may be triggered by a range of factors including body image concerns, perfectionist traits or as a response to adverse experiences. Eating disorders include anorexia nervosa and bulimia nervosa. Signs could include anxiety, depression, sudden loss of appetite, sudden loss of weight or vomiting after food. If you become aware that a student has an eating disorder then this should be referred to the personal tutor. The personal tutor should meet with the student and discuss the need for a referral to specialist services.

PSYCHOSIS

Psychosis occurs when people lose sense of reality and is associated with hallucinations, delusions and confused thinking. Warning signs include lack of motivation, deterioration of personal hygiene, deterioration in the ability to express emotions and impaired communication. They may appear to be anxious and irritable and they may talk to themselves. Their emotions might fluctuate rapidly. They might express suicidal thoughts. Students with psychosis might start to withdraw, lack motivation and demonstrate a declining academic profile. These students will usually require a referral to specialist support services and medication and therapy may be required as a treatment.

SUICIDAL THOUGHTS

The number of student suicides in recent years is a matter of concern and the reasons for these vary across individuals. If you become aware that a student is experiencing suicidal thoughts, demonstrate to them your concerns and explain to them that you are there to help them; they are not alone. Find time to talk to them properly and demonstrate active and reflective listening. Be non-judgemental and demonstrate empathy. Build rapport and use open questions to structure the discussion. Acknowledge to the student the difficulty in talking about sensitive issues. Do not hesitate to use the word 'suicide'. Discuss with the student appropriate coping strategies and connect them with specialist support in the university. Monitor the student carefully.

SUBSTANCE ABUSE

Students might abuse their bodies with a range of substances including drugs, alcohol, tobacco, glue, medication and other substances. Warning signs could include tiredness or disengagement in class, declining attendance or punctuality, declining academic profile, changes in behaviour, mood or personality, and changes to physical characteristics. If you suspect that a student is substance-abusing, you should meet with them to discuss your concerns. If they make a disclosure, you should remain non-judgemental and discuss with them what support can be provided at course-level to enable them to remain on track in their studies. If you are concerned that the student is at risk of harm, you should support the student to self-refer to medical services. You should document your discussion, the advice that you have given and the actions you have taken.

CONDUCT DISORDERS

Conduct disorder is a broad term for a range of behaviours. Students who have oppositional defiant disorder may:

+ lose their temper or get angry;

+ resent others;

+ argue with those in authority positions;

+ refuse to comply with requests or commands from others;

+ annoy others;

+ blame others;

+ be vindictive towards others.

Oppositional defiant disorder does not include aggression, intimidation or violation against others.

Hyperkinetic conduct disorder is now commonly referred to as attention deficit hyperactivity disorder (ADHD). Students in this group may demonstrate the following characteristics:

+ excessive energy or activity;

+ limited attention;

+ lack of perseverance;

+ a tendency to move from activity to activity without completing any task;

+ low self-esteem;

+ delayed motor development;

+ disorganisation.

It is better to respond to the students' behaviour using a non-confrontational approach. You should speak to the student privately to avoid publicly humiliating them. You should remain calm and try to ascertain the factors that might be contributing to the behaviour. In partnership with the student you should agree on goals which the student is able to achieve, and these should be reviewed regularly. You need to maintain a positive approach and it is good practice to ask the student about the steps that you can take to help them.

● Research by the Institute for Public Policy Research (IPPR) found that over the past five years, 94 per cent of universities have experienced a sharp increase in the number of people trying to access support services, with some institutions noticing a threefold increase.

● In 2017/18, 49,265 undergraduates disclosed a mental illness compared to 8,145 in 2007/08.

● In 2017/18, 8,040 postgraduates disclosed a mental illness compared to 1,260 in 2007/08.

● In 2015, 93 male students and 41 female students committed suicide.

● The number of student suicides in England and Wales has increased since 2001.

(www.universitiesuk.ac.uk/policy-and-analysis/reports/Documents/2018/
minding-our-future-starting-conversation-student-mental-health.pdf)

CRITICAL QUESTIONS

+ Why do you think there has been an increase in cases of student mental ill-health?

+ Why do you think the suicide rate is higher for males?

There are growing concerns about the prevalence of depression within adolescent communities. Depression and its effects on university students has received relatively little attention for many years despite universities often reporting an increase in disclosures (Ibrahim et al, 2012). University students are exposed to many factors that increase their vulnerability to depression, and universities must consider these when developing student-support services. These factors include students having their sleeping and eating routines disturbed, experiencing financial pressures, navigating family and relationship changes and discovering new approaches to assessment. Depression has serious potential to impact on students' long-term prospects and relationships, as well as their short-term academic success. The role of universities is therefore crucial if students affected by depression are to be identified and supported.

CASE STUDY

One university in England has introduced a mental health support programme to provide students with access to mental health advisers offering students personalised and tailored support. These advisers liaise with university faculties and departments, including accommodation staff, so that students' issues can be taken into consideration and responded to flexibly. Advisers also emphasise students' rights within existing equality legislation to try and reduce barriers to disclosure. This provides a supportive environment in which students feel comfortable discussing their mental well-being. Offering access to experienced counsellors, this programme also offers students funded referrals to mindfulness and well-being sessions. These are run independently of the university to promote confidence and ensure confidentiality.

- The number of students withdrawing from university with mental health problems has more than trebled in recent years.

- According to Unite Students' Insight Report 2016, students scored 15 per cent and 22 per cent lower than the total UK population on all four well-being measures (life satisfaction, life worthwhile, happiness, low anxiety).

- 71 per cent of higher education institutions monitor lecture attendance of all students, which can be used as an indicator for early intervention.

- 45 per cent of institutions have a student general practitioner based on-site.

- In 33 per cent of institutions, students can access National Health Service mental health practitioners on-site.

(www.universitiesuk.ac.uk/policy-and-analysis/reports/Documents/2018/minding-our-future-starting-conversation-student-mental-health.pdf)

Universities UK and Papyrus (2014) categorised seven key factors likely to increase students' mental distress:

1. media reporting and bias;
2. life transitions;
3. finance worries;
4. pressures to conform academically;
5. social and cultural pressures;
6. the internet and social media;
7. broader issues including uncertainty and insecurity.

Exposure to these factors and pressures increases students' risk of alcohol and drug misuse, self-harm, suicide and wider health and psychological implications including sleep disturbance, mood instability and physical illnesses. For male students, students who are asylum-seekers and refugees, students identifying as LGBTQ+ or students recently affected by bereavement, the risk of harm is even greater. Universities must develop programmes that not only identify and support vulnerable students but do so within an environment that values inclusion throughout.

CASE STUDY

A university has introduced a compulsory module to all its under-graduate degree programmes to encourage students' discussion of issues relating to substance abuse. Each undergraduate programme has been assigned its own substance abuse practitioner who delivers workshops and seminars. These sessions are designed to equip students with the skills and knowledge required to make decisions that support mental health and reduce instances of substance abuse. Educating students on topics including risk management, habits and addictions and social substance abuse, the university has seen a significant decrease in the number of students reporting and disclosing issues related to substance abuse.

SUMMARY

This chapter has outlined the causes of mental ill-health and the prevalence of these within the student community. The common types of mental illness experienced by students have been identified and the warning signs to support you in recognising these have been explained. You have learned about how you can support students with mental health needs and the implications of failing to identify and support vulnerable students. Universities and their staff play a vital role in supporting student well-being and attainment and this support can reduce instances of self-harm, depression and suicide.

CHECKLIST

This chapter has addressed:

✓ the causes of mental ill-health and the increasing prevalence of these within student and higher education communities;

✓ the role of higher education institutions in identifying and supporting students with vulnerabilities;

✓ the value of creating cultures and environments which support students and encourage disclosure without fear of judgement or failure.

FURTHER READING

Benas, N and Hart, M (2017) *Mental Health Emergencies*.
New York: Hatherleigh Press.

✚ CHAPTER 4

SUPPORTING STUDENT MENTAL HEALTH

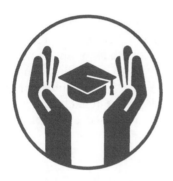

PROFESSIONAL LINKS

This chapter addresses the following:

Houghton, A M and Anderson, J (2017) *Embedding Mental Wellbeing in the Curriculum: Maximising Success in Higher Education*. Higher Education Academy.

CHAPTER OBJECTIVES

After reading this chapter you will understand:

+ the elements of the whole-institution approach to mental health;

+ the roles of different service providers in the university.

INTRODUCTION

This chapter will introduce you to an institution-wide approach to student mental health. An institution-wide approach focuses on developing approaches that enable all students and staff to be mentally healthy. It is an approach that aims to meet the needs of all, and it seeks to be preventative, thus reducing the number of students who demonstrate signs of mental ill-health. This chapter will take you through the institution-wide approach and discuss the roles and responsibilities of different services.

DEVELOPING AN INSTITUTION-WIDE STRATEGY FOR MENTAL HEALTH

A university-wide framework for mental health should be developed through a process of consultation with key stakeholders. These include teaching and support staff, students, the student union, institutional leaders and managers, and external service providers such as the National Health Service. A task and finish group should be established to develop the framework.

INSTITUTIONAL LEADERSHIP

The senior leadership team in the institution need to demonstrate their strategic commitment to promoting positive mental health in students and staff. This commitment also needs to be supported by deans of faculties, heads of schools and departments and course leaders. Examples of activities that might support the development of mentally healthy cultures for students and staff include:

+ developing a well-being/mental health policy;

+ itemising mental health as a standing agenda item on committee minutes;

+ reviewing new policies through a well-being and mental health lens prior to implementation;

+ flexible working policies, including opportunities for home working;

+ well-being events for staff;

+ reducing work overload in relation to student assessment;

+ reducing staff time spent in committee meetings;

+ reducing bureaucracy for staff through removing bureaucratic tasks;

+ clear and fair staff promotion policies;

+ regular opportunities for staff and students to discuss the extent to which they feel that their well-being is supported.

CRITICAL QUESTIONS

+ What other ways can you think of for institutional leaders to demonstrate a commitment to promoting positive mental health?

+ What strategies might need to be in place to support the mental health of institutional leaders?

CAMPUS CLIMATE AND ETHOS

The campus climate and ethos are critical to the development of positive mental health in students and staff. Various factors contribute to campus climate. There needs to be a visible indicator around the campus that demonstrates that staff and student diversity are valued and celebrated. Celebration events can be a powerful signal that disability and social, cultural, political, gender and sexual diversity are valued. Outward-facing resources including course publicity materials, websites and social media need to reflect this commitment to diversity. The environment should be adapted to cater for the needs of students with physical disabilities. The way in which staff and students communicate sends out powerful signals about whether all individuals are valued.

Campus climate also extends beyond environmental factors to include the extent to which the campus climate engenders a sense of belonging and connectedness. Staff and students who do not experience a sense of belonging and do not feel connected to the institution are less likely to remain at the institution. Additionally, students who do not experience a sense of belonging are more likely to achieve lower academic outcomes than those who feel connected to the institution.

CRITICAL QUESTIONS

+ What other factors contribute to a positive campus climate?

+ What factors contribute to a negative campus climate?

CURRICULUM, TEACHING AND LEARNING

Within the whole-institution approach, the curriculum is designed to promote positive mental health in students. One way of addressing this in higher education is to integrate the relevant skills and knowledge into existing course content and to design assessment tasks that enable students to develop these skills and knowledge. An example of this is to develop resilience skills in each taught module so that student resilience increases. Improved resilience can be a protective factor against mental ill-health. Students can learn about aspects of mental health within modules where this has relevance. For example, psychology students can be introduced to psychological perspectives on mental health. Sociology students can learn about the effects of social environments on people's mental health. Art students can use artistic media to develop their own representations of mental health and mental illness. History students can learn about historical perspectives on mental illness.

CRITICAL QUESTIONS

+ What other examples can you generate of integrating mental health through the taught curriculum in higher education?

+ What various forms of resilience do students and staff need to develop in higher education?

Approaches to assessment should be carefully designed to min-imise student and staff workload, which can result in stress. Teaching sessions should be designed so that students can study in emotionally safe and democratic learning environments. Teaching should be inclu-sive and teaching staff will need to consider how barriers to learning, participation and achievement will be removed for students with spe-cific needs, such as those with disabilities.

STUDENT AND STAFF VOICE

Providing students and staff with a voice is empowering and engenders a sense of belonging. Course leaders and module leaders should include students in planning and designing learning content. This ensures that students are learning about subject-specific aspects of development which they perceive as important. Involving students in designing assessment tasks is also a good way of providing them with ownership of their courses. Often lecturers ask students for feedback about their experiences but rarely are students consulted about course design and assessment. Acting on student feedback is also important and many institutions now provide students with feedback on how their suggestions have been acted upon, for example using strategies such as 'you said, we did'.

Institutional leaders should consult staff about the process of change. Change is essential in all organisations to ensure that the service is current but when change is imposed from those in positions of power without con-sultation, this can be demoralising and result in staff resistance.

CRITICAL QUESTIONS

+ What other strategies might be adopted to promote student voice?
+ When might student voice lead to tokenism?

STAFF DEVELOPMENT

This book has emphasised that mental health is everyone's respon-sibility within a higher education institution. It is therefore important that staff and students can identify the signs and symptoms of mental ill-health. An institution-wide commitment to professional learning will ensure that people with mental ill-health can get the right support rapidly. Many institutions now require specific staff to undertake training courses that enable them to understand the risk factors, types of mental ill-health and strategies for supporting people with mental health needs. While it is beneficial for all staff to undertake professional learning in mental health, this might not be feasible within a large institution and leaders and managers will need to decide which staff will participate in these opportunities. Staff with student-facing responsibilities such as teaching staff and staff in support roles should be given priority. Additionally, some universities are now developing the role of student mental health champions. This is further explained in the case study below. These students will need to be provided with opportunities to undertake professional learning in mental health.

CASE STUDY

A university developed the role of student mental health champion. Students were required to formally apply for the role and following application there was an interview process. Students who were accepted to be champions were paid for the hours they spent undertaking the role. All champions subsequently completed a professional learning course on mental health which lasted two days. The course included an assessment task which needed to be passed before students could undertake the role. The champions received a certificate for successfully passing the course.

Once the training was successfully completed, the champions were linked to schools and departments. Their role was to be a friendly 'listening ear' to other students with specific mental health needs. The champions advertised their role to students across the school or department. They ran a weekly one-to-one surgery which was managed through an online booking system. In addition, the champions ran a specific weekly timetabled slot where they could provide support to other students via instant messaging software. This allowed the service users to maintain anonymity. Finally, the champions provided support to students who could not attend the face-to-face surgery via telephone or video conferencing.

The scheme was a huge success. The user feedback was extremely positive, and students commented that they preferred to speak to a peer rather than to a member of staff.

CRITICAL QUESTIONS

+ What criteria would you develop to support the recruitment of student mental health champions?

+ Do the champions need to be experts in all types of mental ill-health?

+ What are the implications for student confidentiality in schemes such as this?

+ When would it be appropriate for student champions to refer cases to specialist support?

+ Do you think that the champions need to have personal experiences of mental ill-health to enable them to carry out their role?

+ What are the attributes of a good student champion?

Peer mentoring is neither a new concept, nor is it specific to the United Kingdom. It was first employed in the United States in the 1970s, and it has been used in countries such as Canada and Australia since the 1980s. Peer mentoring is now used widely in several countries across the world, including the UK, Italy, Spain, Finland, Japan, New Zealand, Saudi Arabia, Norway, the Netherlands and South Africa (Coleman et al, 2017). Research on its effectiveness is inconclusive, largely because a wide range of models exist, which are operationalised differently, and programmes are established to measure a variety of outcomes (Coleman et al, 2017). Programmes of peer support can include one-to-one, group and online support. While the evidence on the effectiveness of peer-mentoring schemes is largely inconclusive (Weare and Nind, 2011), research suggests that there are several key characteristics of effective peer support programmes, specifically those that focus on mental health and well-being. First, commitment from senior leaders in the institution is essential to the success of programmes (Houlston and Smith, 2009). Second, the programme needs to be led and managed by a dedicated member of staff, who can monitor the quality of the programme, ensure that it is running smoothly and provide support to the peer mentors as well as the mentees (James, 2011). Third, effective marketing of the scheme and celebration events for participants which include rewards can give the scheme status and overcome stigma (MBF, 2011).

IDENTIFYING NEED AND MONITORING IMPACT

Higher education institutions need to develop approaches to evaluate the impact of their mental health provision. In schemes such as the student mental health champion scheme, the university made a financial investment in the service. The university will need to evaluate this provision regularly to see if it is providing good value for money. Collecting anonymous service-user feedback is a particularly effective way of evaluating the provision and this can be collated in a short report and given to the Strategic Board. Additionally, in this instance it is also useful to collect some generic quantitative information. This might include:

+ the number of appointments over time;

+ demographic information about service users, including gender, ethnicity, disability and age;

+ numbers of referrals to central support services;

+ anonymous data to capture the impact of the service on student attendance, progression and retention.

Universal provision may also be provided by the student union through the development of clubs and societies that exist to support students' personal development. Sports teams and groups that focus on other forms of physical activity are good examples of providing a service which enhances student well-being through the social connections that are formed and the strong positive correlation between physical activity and mental health. Other societies exist to improve students' well-being, provide opportunities for personal and social development and enable students to develop new interests and skills. Examples include outdoor activities, reading groups, debating societies, LGBTQ+ societies and film clubs. These opportunities are available to all students and they can impact positively on students' mental health. Evaluating the impact of this provision is crucial and the perspectives of users are critical to inform future development. Monitoring levels of participation and the demographic profiles of users is an important way of analysing whether specific groups of students are not participating in the opportunities. The barriers to participation can then be identified through consultation with non-users.

TARGETED SUPPORT

Higher education providers offer a range of specialist services that allow students to access specialist support. Examples of services include counselling, disability support, accommodation support, academic skills support, careers advice and financial support. Personal tutors need to know when to refer students for specialist targeted support and some students will self-refer to these services. These services may carry out a detailed assessment of the student's needs and then provide a programme of intervention to address the needs of the student. Each service will develop mechanisms for monitoring the impact of the service. Reports of impact should focus less on describing the range of support that is available and focus more on the impact that the service has had on student attendance, retention, progression and well-being.

WORKING IN PARTNERSHIP

Higher education institutions, and specifically senior managers, should work in partnership with a range of services that may also be based on campus to support students' mental health. These may include:

+ health services;

+ police;

+ student union;

+ adult social care services;

+ support workers employed through disability funding.

Students in higher education are adults and therefore referrals to specialist services should only be made with student consent. There are exceptions to this; for example, if the student is at risk of significant harm. Students may already be accessing specialist support from other professionals (such as social workers, medical professionals, counsellors or therapists). They are not required to inform the university of this support, but they may choose to do so.

A 2012 survey of more than 5,500 students found that:

- 81 per cent thought counselling had helped them stay in higher education;

- 79 per cent thought it helped them improve their academic work;

- 78 per cent thought it helped them develop skills useful for obtaining employment.

(Patti Wallace, The Impact of Counselling on Academic Outcomes: The Student Perspective, *British Association of Counselling and Psychotherapy*, November 2012)

Recent discourse in higher education has positioned students as consumers rather than willing learners (Molesworth et al, 2009). There has been an emphasis on neo-liberalist principles (Saunders, 2011), which has emphasised student satisfaction, value for money (Carey, 2013), competition and outcomes for students. Within this *'consumerist paradigm'* (Carey, 2013, p 251), the student is rebranded as a client of the university. In the UK, student satisfaction is measured through the National Student Survey, which reinforces a consumerist focus on satisfaction (Gibbs, 2010) rather than focusing on students' perspectives on engagement. This focus on consumerism assumes that students make purchasing decisions based on how satisfied they are with the services they receive. Universities see their students as sources of income and use this assumption to marketise the services they offer (Carey, 2013). However, there is evidence to suggest that while students may sometimes act as customers, this is not their prime motivation (Woodall et al, 2012).

The Student as Producer framework situates the learning experience as a co-production between students and their universities (Carey, 2013). It represents a direct challenge to managerialism (McCulloch, 2009) and consumerist principles and provides students with significant opportunities to take ownership of their curriculum and learning (Neary, 2010). The model essentially positions students as social agents; they are viewed as capable and confident and able to participate equally with lecturers in aspects such as curriculum design and knowledge generation. Within this framework, students are not only required to provide feedback on their experiences, they are required to actively engage in offering solutions to problems that they have identified. Rather than viewing students as passive recipients of knowledge, students are positioned as active producers of knowledge. The process of learning is given greater significance than the products of learning. Through active engagement in this model, students learn to listen to offers, empathise, challenge and negotiate. As they are required to take responsibility for their own education, the power imbalance between lecturers and students is eradicated.

Within this model, students are actively engaged in designing curricula and assessment tasks. They are given responsibility for knowledge generation and great emphasis is placed on collaborative group tasks in which students investigate a problem or a theme and then disseminate their findings.

The Student as Producer framework can potentially create a *rhizomatic* learning environment (Coley et al, 2012) in which educators and students weave away alongside one another in a non-hierarchical relationship. Within a rhizomatic model students can weave their own learning pathways. There is a sense of connectivity between students and between students and educators and the relationships between them are equal. Within a rhizomatic structure there are no limits to achievement. The learner is positioned as ever-growing, ever-moving, and the role of the educator is reframed as a facilitator of learning rather than a knowledge-transmitter. The students become experts in their own learning – they shape and reshape their curriculum and they take responsibility for generating knowledge. This represents a worldwide movement of scholars and students against the neo-liberalist principles that higher education has unquestioningly embraced. The University of Lincoln is leading the sector in this area and in doing so is challenging the '*intellectual vandalism*' (Neary, 2012, p 2) caused by the increasing privatisation of higher education.

A 2016 Unite survey found that, among students who had strongly considered withdrawing from their higher education course:

- 76 per cent reported feeling stressed or worried;
- 46 per cent reported feeling down or depressed;
- 43 per cent reported feeling isolated or lonely.

(Unite Students Insight Report, 2016, www.unitestudents.com/about-us/insightreport/2016-full-report)

CASE STUDY

One university has introduced several initiatives to build students' resilience and improve well-being throughout the student body. These initiatives include:

+ distributing introductory materials to support transition;

+ a 24-hour text messaging service connecting students with counsellors and mental health practitioners;

+ creating healthy living toolkits to support students' life skills;

+ providing job shop carousels to support students who have had to leave employment to pursue their higher education study;

+ delivering workshops to address factors contributing to stress and anxiety;

+ supporting students in differentiating between stressful experiences that may be ordinary and those that may be more serious;

+ activities to support communication and relationships for students living on campus;

+ timetabling flexibility to support students with mental ill-health who are likely to benefit from opportunities to visit friends and family in their home towns;

+ progress tutorials to involve friends, tutors and parents in supporting students who are struggling either socially or academically.

SUMMARY

This chapter has explored the importance of institutions developing holistic approaches to supporting mental health. The value of these approaches has been explained in the context of supporting both staff and students. The roles and responsibilities of internal and external support services have been identified. This chapter has also highlighted the difference between preventative approaches and reactive approaches and the importance of both has been considered in ensuring all stakeholders are mentally healthy.

CHECKLIST

This chapter has addressed:

✓ strategies to prevent the onset of mental ill-health in students;

✓ the importance of institution-wide approaches in supporting
the mental health of staff and students;

✓ the roles and responsibilities of internal and external support
services and the need for these organisations to work
together.

FURTHER READING

Iarovici, D (2014), *Mental Health Issues and the University Student.*
Baltimore, MD: Johns Hopkins University Press.

✚ CHAPTER 5

SUPPORTING VULNERABLE STUDENTS AT UNIVERSITY

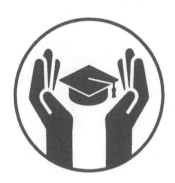

PROFESSIONAL LINKS

This chapter addresses the following:

The 2010 Equality Act places a legal duty on all higher education institutions to ensure that there is no direct or indirect direct discrimination against students with protected characteristics. Institutions must be able to demonstrate that reasonable adjustments have been applied to ensure that students with protected characteristics experience equality of opportunity.

CHAPTER OBJECTIVES

After reading this chapter you will understand:

+ some of the barriers to learning, participation and achievement experienced by specific groups of students;

+ strategies to address these barriers.

INTRODUCTION

Higher education institutions are increasingly demonstrating a commitment to recruiting a diverse student body. This ensures that institutions reflect the communities and societies in which students live and enables universities to advance social justice. However, with this commitment comes a responsibility to ensure that students with diverse needs are adequately supported so that they experience equality of opportunity. The Equality Act (2010) makes it illegal for public institutions to discriminate against people on the basis of:

+ age;

+ disability;

+ gender reassignment;

+ marriage and civil partnership;

+ pregnancy and maternity;

+ race;

+ religion or belief;

+ sex;

+ sexual orientation.

This protection from discrimination affects all aspects of the student lifecycle from gaining entry to the institution through to graduation. Higher education institutions are not allowed to discriminate against students in the admissions process on the basis of these characteristics. Approaches to learning and teaching must ensure that all students are able to participate in the process of learning. In addition, adjustments should be made to assessment processes so that students with protected characteristics are given the same chances of achieving as other students.

This chapter focuses on specific groups of students. You will learn about the barriers to learning, participation and achievement that may result in mental ill-health for specific groups of students and you will be introduced to strategies for addressing these barriers. As you read this chapter it is worth remembering that students are individuals. While this chapter uses categories to describe characteristics of students, no two students will present an identical profile; they have different needs and respond to educational interventions differently.

SUPPORTING STUDENTS WITH AUTISM

Students with a diagnosis of autistic spectrum conditions may find aspects of university life challenging. Autism is a lifelong developmental condition that affects the way individuals interact and communicate socially with others. The groundbreaking work of Lorna Wing in the 1980s has significantly shaped our understanding of autism. Wing identified that individuals on the autistic spectrum experience three main areas of difficulty. These are:

+ social interaction;

+ social communication;

+ inflexibility of thought.

These difficulties are evident to a greater or lesser extent in all individuals who are diagnosed with autistic spectrum conditions. Difficulties with social interaction mean that navigating the campus environment can be stressful for students with autism. They might feel anxious in social places around the campus or in classrooms where they will be expected to work in groups or pairs. They might struggle to cope with group tasks or group assessments and they may find it stressful in noisy and bright environments due to sensory sensitivities.

Difficulties with social communication are not usually related to language or vocabulary use in students with autism. Often their language and vocabulary skills are highly developed because most will have high-functioning autism (or Asperger's). The difficulties lie in understanding the social rules of communication. These include verbal and non-verbal skills including turn taking, eye contact, gesture, facial expression, knowing when to take pauses and building on what others have said. The deficit is related to understanding the use of language for communication.

Students with autism tend to demonstrate rigid thought processes. They may struggle with sudden changes to routines. They may develop an obsession with punctuality and often have a need for a consistent routine. This can make aspects of university life extremely challenging, particularly when lectures do not start on time or are cancelled or there are unexpected changes to rooms, deadlines or course design.

It is important that students with autism are adequately supported right from the start of their student lifecycle. Consideration should be given to facilitating their transition to university. Students with autism may need to visit the campus several times to familiarise themselves with the physical layout of the campus and any teaching spaces. It is a good idea for them to meet key staff before they start university. If they are moving away from home for the first time, it might be the first time they have been required to cope without the support of family members. Meeting new people in university accommodation can be stressful and living independently for the first time, managing their self-care, finances and time, can be challenging.

It is important for students with autism to meet their personal tutor as soon as possible. If you are a personal tutor you will need to check that all entitled support is in place right from the start. You should talk to the student about what they find difficult and what support they think they need to enable them to thrive, particularly in relation to their learning and modifications to assessment tasks. You should meet with them very regularly at the start of their course to ascertain how well they are settling in and to find out if they need additional support. You should communicate any concerns, with student consent, to relevant staff. You might need to support them in managing their unstructured time. Typically, higher education study includes significant self-directed study time and students with autism may find this challenging. You can support them in planning how they might use this time.

If you are a lecturer you should ensure that timetable changes are kept to a minimum. If there needs to be changes to the timetable you should communicate these to the students in advance so that they are prepared. Sudden changes to times and rooms can cause students with autism to experience stress and anxiety. You should also consider the following:

+ providing handouts in advance through the virtual learning platform;

+ providing assessment briefs that explain the task clearly and explicitly state what students need to do to achieve specific grades;

+ allowing students to remove themselves from classrooms if they need to go to a quiet space;

+ reducing sensory overload in teaching spaces;

+ using visual strategies in your teaching;

+ providing additional support to enable students with autism to complete group tasks.

These strategies will alleviate stress and anxiety and enable students with autism to thrive.

CRITICAL QUESTIONS

+ Do you think these strategies would be useful for all students? Explain your answer.

+ What adjustments might be needed to the physical environment of the campus to facilitate a sense of belonging for autistic students?

+ What contribution can university leaders and managers make to support students with autism, specifically in relation to the physical environment of the campus and to teaching, learning and assessment?

Approximately 40 per cent of people with autism have symptoms of at least one anxiety disorder at any time, compared with up to 15 per cent in the general population.

(www.autism.org.uk/about/health/mental-health.aspx)

According to Fabri, Andrews and Pukki (2013, p 13):

There is evidence that some students know they are autistic but choose not to declare it ... This can be for a variety of reasons including not identifying as disabled, believing they are not entitled to support or wanting to fit in with their peers. Further, a large number of students with an autism spectrum condition have not been diagnosed by the time they start university, especially female and gender non-conforming students.

SUPPORTING LGBTQ+ STUDENTS

Students who identify as LGBTQ+ need to experience a sense of belonging to their institutions. They have a right to feel respected and institutions have a legal duty to protect them from direct or indirect discrimination. Some universities now demonstrate a visible commitment to the LGBTQ+ community through anti-homophobic, anti-biphobic and anti-transphobic signs, and some display the LGBTQ+ flags. In some universities, staff may wear rainbow lanyards to demonstrate a visible commitment to LGBTQ+ inclusion. Some student unions are working tirelessly to challenge homophobia in sport and to provide inclusive physical activities. Many universities now show a visible presence at LGBTQ+ events such as Pride. However, while these approaches have good intentions, they only offer a surface-level response to inclusion. Some forms of discrimination and prejudice may be subtle rather than overt. Higher education managers should ensure that all staff have undertaken training in subconscious bias so that students who identify as LGBTQ+ are not marginalised.

In the United States, research suggests that homophobia on campus is endemic and there is evidence of physical violence and verbal harassment (Ellis, 2009). This has resulted in a *climate of fear* (Ellis, 2009, p 727) in which students do not feel comfortable disclosing their sexual identity. While violence and verbal harassment is less common on campuses in the UK, research has found that fears relating to prejudice and discrimination impacted negatively on levels of 'outness' in universities (Formby, 2012, 2013, 2015). Some LGBTQ+ students may negotiate their sexual identity by passing off as heterosexual or by covering up their sexuality if the campus climate does not foster a sense of belonging.

One example of fostering a culture of deep inclusion for LGBTQ+ students is through inclusive curriculum design. Keenan (2014) has emphasised the invisibility of LGBTQ+ issues in the higher education curriculum, supporting earlier research by Ellis (2009). This can result in marginalisation, and curriculum invisibility is worse for transgender students who have reported a lack of trans experiences and trans history reflected in their curriculum (McKinney, 2005; Metro, 2014; NUS, 2014). Another example relates to the organisation of physical space on the campus and some institutions now provide safe social spaces on campus for LGBTQ+ students to meet and gender-neutral toilets throughout university buildings.

If you are a personal tutor you should meet with students who identify as LGBTQ+ regularly to check that they are not experiencing prejudice or discrimination, either on campus or in student accommodation. You will also need to monitor their attendance and progress. You should consider making a referral to counselling, with student consent, if a student is presenting with mental health difficulties. However, it is important to remember that a standard response of making a referral to student counselling is not appropriate because it may be interpreted negatively by the student.

If you are a lecturer you have a legal duty to challenge bullying in classrooms, including subtle forms of bullying such as segregation, 'knowing' looks, smiles and laughs in the absence of verbal comments. You should be prepared to use students' preferred pronouns and pre-ferred names for those who identify as non-gender-conforming. Finding opportunities to include LGBTQ+ issues into the curriculum is an effective way of engendering a sense of belonging. Effective ways of doing this include:

+ referring to famous role models within the subject who identify as LGBTQ+;

+ including opportunities to study LGBTQ+ history;

+ studying patterns of LGBTQ+ migration in geography;

+ opportunities to learn about LGBTQ+ prejudice and discrimination in sociology;

+ discussing homophobia in sport in sports studies course;

+ considering LGBTQ+ news articles in journalism courses;

+ including LGBTQ+ equality in the workplace in business management courses;

+ including psychological perspectives in psychology courses in relation to individuals who identify as LGBTQ+;

+ studying LGBTQ+ authors and texts in English;

+ discussing religious perspectives on LGBTQ+ issues in theology courses;

+ including content on LGBTQ+ issues in education and teacher training courses.

Research indicates that for students who identify as LGBTQ+, perceptions of safety, acceptance and tolerance (Formby, 2014) are important factors that influence university choice-making. Choice of university for students who identify as LGBTQ+ may be influenced by previous negative experience at school (Formby, 2014, 2015). They may choose a university which they perceive to offer a safe space so that previous experiences of bullying, prejudice and harassment are not repeated. Perceptions of safety can also be influenced by scene size and vibrancy. Universities with large and vibrant gay scenes nearby are perceived to be more tolerant and supportive and offer safe spaces for those who identify as LGBTQ+ (Epstein et al, 2003; Formby, 2015; Taulke-Johnson, 2010; Valentine et al, 2009). This mirrors broader research about LGBTQ+ migration, which has demonstrated how urban locations with large scenes tend to attract migrants from the gay community (Browne, 2008; Formby, 2012; Valentine et al, 2003; Weeks et al, 2001). Research has found that students who identify as LGBTQ+ may desire to escape from heterosexist and homophobic home communities that have '*strictly regulated boundaries of acceptable (ie heterosexual) behaviour*' (Taulke-Johnson, 2010, p 256).

CRITICAL QUESTIONS

+ As a lecturer, how might you embed LGBTQ+ inclusion into your curriculum?

+ What factors would help to create a positive campus climate for students who identify as LGBTQ+?

SUPPORTING STUDENTS WHO ARE CARE LEAVERS

Students who leave the care of local authorities or foster care are under-represented in universities. Their previous experiences of the care and education systems may mean that these students arrive at university with mental ill-health. The reasons why they were placed in care will vary across individuals and this is not a question you should ask. However, students may be happy to disclose this information to people they trust. Building effective relationships with care leavers is essential so that they develop trust. This is more easily achieved through building confidence, self-esteem and self-belief. Care leavers may not have had the opportunity to develop secure attachments with their primary carers and this can impact on their psychological development. Providing them with a named contact who they can meet regularly for support is one way of enabling attachments.

CRITICAL QUESTIONS

+ What are the implications for personal tutors in relation to supporting students who have left care?
+ What are the implications for teaching staff?
+ Why do you think there is an under-representation of students who are care leavers in higher education?

CASE STUDY

Several universities across the United Kingdom have developed systems to support care leavers considering, applying to and studying within higher education. One of these universities has established a support group staffed by university counsellors and advisers to support care leavers. The support group offers its services prior to, during and after a student's study and establishes first contact with students following the submission of a UCAS application. Advisers are each allocated to specific students and provide advice on logistics and transport, finance and bursary support, and accommodation applications. Applications for each of these services are given priority status if care leavers have been unable to apply before a deadline because of reasons related to personal circumstances.

6 per cent of those looked after or leaving care in England pursue higher education compared to 40 per cent of the wider population.

2 per cent of those looked after or leaving care in Scotland pursue higher education compared to 40 per cent of the wider population.

(www.ucas.com/file/4996/download?token=YI9B1Wwh)

69

SUPPORTING STUDENTS WITH DISABILITIES

Students with disabilities are an under-represented group in higher education. Specific needs may include:

+ cognition and learning needs;

+ sensory and physical impairment;

+ social, emotional and mental health needs;

+ communication and language needs.

Many students with disabilities will have undertaken an assessment with the disability support team prior to starting on their course. If a personal learning plan has been issued to teaching staff and course leaders, this should be reviewed, discussed with the student and implemented. Some students have undiagnosed needs when they enter higher education and may need to be encouraged to undertake a formal assessment by the disability support team. Personal tutors play a crucial role in initiating discussions with the student about the support they think they will need. Teaching staff should aim to deliver high-quality inclusive teaching to maximise opportunities for participation. Barriers to learning should be identified and removed. Clear assignment briefs, a well-designed and up-to-date virtual learning platform and opportunities for formative assessment will help to ensure that students with disabilities have access to equality of opportunity. Course leaders and personal tutors should review their progress regularly and maintain ongoing discussions with the student about further adaptations that will facilitate their inclusion.

If disabled students are required to undertake professional placements, the student's permission must be sought before their disability is disclosed to the placement provider. Universities should ensure that reasonable adjustments are in place to enable the student to complete the placement successfully. If the student is happy for you to disclose their disability to a placement provider, a joint meeting with a university representative, the student and a placement representative is a useful way of identifying what reasonable adjustments might be necessary to enable the student to complete the placement successfully. This meeting should ideally take place in advance of a placement starting.

SUPPORTING INTERNATIONAL STUDENTS

International students are students who choose to study in the UK from other countries. They experience multiple transitions. These include:

+ social transitions – meeting new people, forming new friendships;

+ geographical transitions – adapting to a new country, town, or city and community;

+ academic transitions – adapting to different approaches to teaching, learning and assessment;

+ psychological transitions – adapting to a new identity as an international student;

+ cultural transitions – adapting to new cultural norms that may sharply contrast with those in their home country;

+ workplace transitions – adapting to culturally different expectations in the workplace for those students who need to find part-time work to subsidise their studies.

Moving to a new country can be exciting and stressful and it can impact on students' mental health. If you teach international students or if you are a personal tutor, it is useful to develop your cultural knowledge so that you understand the cultural values that these students may arrive with. It is useful to research a little about the country where these students come from so that you can connect with them and begin to foster a sense of belonging. Demonstrating an awareness of the cultural values, customs and current affairs of a student's home country will demonstrate that you are interested in where they have come from.

Some international students may expect a very didactic approach to teaching. They may be used to traditional transmission models of teaching where the lecturer imparts knowledge to a passive group of students. Some international students develop a belief that they are not learning anything because their lecturer is not teaching them everything that they need to know. They may initially struggle to see the relevance of group tasks and self-directed study. Some will relish the more liberal and democratic style of teaching.

All international students are required to demonstrate that they are attending their courses in order to fulfil their visa requirements. If you are a course leader or personal tutor, you will need to monitor their attendance

71

very carefully and you will be required to report on this regularly during the academic year. Poor attendance can lead to visas being retracted.

If you are responsible for teaching international students, you can support their inclusion by:

+ expressing yourself in lectures and seminars with clarity;

+ using visuals in your teaching to support your explanations;

+ providing very clear assignment briefs so that students have clarity on the task they need to complete;

+ explaining UK-specific subject content;

+ drawing on the cultural, social and political perspectives from their 'home' context in your teaching;

+ using their names in class;

+ encouraging UK and non-UK students to work together in mixed groups so that silos do not form.

International students may develop mental ill-health for a variety of reasons. They may develop homesickness. If there is political conflict in their home country they may be anxious about the safety of family members and friends. They may lack confidence in their academic writing and they may need academic support from academic skills tutors. They may struggle with managing unstructured time when they are not on campus and they may feel isolated in their accommodation.

CRITICAL QUESTIONS

+ Why is cultural sensitivity important when working with international students?

+ How might you internationalise the curriculum content in your discipline?

CASE STUDY

To ensure the academic success and engagement of international students, one university has introduced a staff training course that must be taken by all university staff once per year. This training course is used to reinforce the university's commitment to equality and diversity and reminds staff of the university's policies regarding the recruitment and admission of international students. This university has also introduced an online chat service that international students can use, prior to application, to discuss the typical cost of living and access support with visa applications. By ensuring that key documents are printed in many languages, international students can share important information with non-English speaking parents, encouraging family buy-in and influencing students' aspirations.

SUPPORTING STUDENTS WHO ARE CARERS

Some students arrive at university with family caring commitments. They might be looking after younger siblings or parents who have ill-health. They will need to balance their academic studies alongside their family commitments and this can be stressful. In addition, if they have ill family members, they may be experiencing signs of anxiety. University staff need to be supportive and flexible about attendance, punctuality and assessment deadlines to enable these students to have equality of opportunity. Personal tutors should meet regularly with these students to monitor their progress and their well-being. Tutors should ensure that the virtual learning platform includes up-to-date content on lectures and seminars, including live recordings of lectures and video podcasts of assessment briefs. Tutors should also be prepared to conduct tutorials via video conferencing if the student is unable to attend campus.

SUMMARY

This chapter has identified the barriers to learning, participation and achievement facing specific groups of students including those with autism, those identifying as LGBTQ+, those with disabilities and those applying as an international student. Strategies to address some of the barriers facing these students have been suggested and the legal protections available have been made clear. Strategies to engage and support care leavers and carers have been discussed and a best practice case study illustrates and illuminates the valuable role universities play in supporting students from all backgrounds.

CHECKLIST

This chapter has addressed:

✓ the barriers to learning, participation and achievement facing students from a range of diverse backgrounds and with varying needs;

✓ strategies to overcome students' barriers and the role universities play in ensuring and promoting inclusive environments for all students;

✓ the legislative protections in place and the importance to higher education institutions of understanding, implementing and complying with these.

FURTHER READING

Grace, S and Gravestock, P (2008) *Inclusion and Diversity: Meeting the Needs of All Students*. London: Routledge.

CHAPTER 6

SUPPORTING TRANSITIONS THROUGH HIGHER EDUCATION

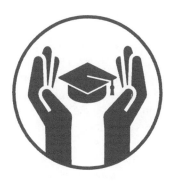

PROFESSIONAL LINKS

This chapter addresses the following:

The Teaching Excellence Framework emphasises the need for higher education institutions to retain students and to support them in gaining graduate employment.

CHAPTER OBJECTIVES

After reading this chapter you will understand:

+ theoretical perspectives on transition through higher education;

+ practical implications for transition beyond the first year of study;

+ strategies for supporting transitions into professional contexts.

INTRODUCTION

This chapter examines student transitions throughout higher education and the implications of these for students' mental health. As students progress through their studies they will experience a variety of challenges, including the increased demands of higher-level academic study. In addition, they may experience social, geographical and psychological transitions that can impact on their mental health. This chapter provides you with practical advice on how you can support students through these transitions to minimise any detrimental impact on their mental health. Theoretical perspectives on transition are addressed and case studies of effective practice illustrate what institutions can do to facilitate smooth transitions.

THEORETICAL PERSPECTIVES ON TRANSITION

This section revisits some of the theoretical perspectives on student transition that were presented in Chapter 1. Specifically, transition as induction, development and becoming will be addressed. Critical questions are included to enable you to consider the implications of each of these theoretical perspectives on students' mental health.

THE IMPORTANCE OF TRANSITION

Research on contemporary student transitions forms part of a broader body of work that focuses on life transitions, although the work on life transitions is dominated by an interest in student transitions (Ingram et al, 2009). Interest in student transitions has increased in the past three decades (Bauman, 2001; Field, 2010; Giddens, 1990), although research on life transitions is still largely underdeveloped (Ingram et al, 2009).

Interest in student transitions has increased, partly due to the expansion of higher education, particularly in the UK, over the past two decades (Gale and Parker, 2014). The expansion of higher education has led to researchers emphasising the importance of transition (Heirdsfield et al, 2008; Hultberg et al, 2009; Kift et al, 2010). Policy imperatives have focused on increasing the numbers of students in higher education from diverse backgrounds and improving student engagement and retention. While the massification of higher education is not new, the introduction of the Teaching Excellence Framework in the UK in 2015 has signalled a clear policy commitment to increasing access to higher education for students from under-represented groups, including those from areas of social deprivation and minority ethnic backgrounds. Institutions that succeed in recruiting and retaining these students are rewarded for their efforts in relation to this policy priority. Research on student transitions in higher education has progressed beyond its original focus on access (Belyakov et al, 2009; Gale and Parker, 2014) to increased emphasis on student outcomes (Osborne and Gallacher, 2007). Consequently, the emphasis has shifted towards transitions throughout an undergraduate programme rather than focusing solely on the first year of undergraduate study (Gale and Parker, 2014).

Despite the emphasis on student transition Ecclestone, Biesta and Hughes (2010, p 5) have stated that *'there is no agreed upon definition of what constitutes a transition'*. It is also interesting that in much of the research the concept of transition is rarely critically interrogated or even considered (Gale and Parker, 2014). Without a clear understanding of what constitutes a transition, it is difficult for higher education practitioners to recognise transitions or to know how to support students when they experience transitions. According to Worth:

Many researchers have discussed how transitions have changed – how they no longer follow a traditional linear path – but much of this research on youth transitions does not really provide an alternative to the linear path.

(Worth, 2009, p 1051)

Traditionally, transition has been defined as *'a fixed turning point which takes place at a preordained time and in a certain place'* (Quinn, 2010, p 122). However, Gale and Parker (2014, p 737) define transition as *'the capability to navigate change'*. This shifts the emphasis away from focusing on the process of change over time (Colley, 2007) to an emphasis on students' capabilities to navigate and negotiate the process of change. Other researchers have emphasised transition as a *multidimensional* process, which takes place over time (Lent et al, 2007). If transition is understood through a capability framework it is important to consider agency and structure, both of which will influence how effectively an individual can navigate the change (Ecclestone, 2009; Ecclestone et al, 2010). While individual agency can be influenced by personal aspirations (Sellar and Gale, 2011; Smith, 2009), university structures can facilitate or impede an individual's capacity to navigate change. In higher education, the policies of the institution, the curriculum that students study and the assessment process to which they are subjected form structural factors that can facilitate or restrict personal agency. University policies which emphasise institutional commitments to equality and diversity may not support a smooth transition if students do not *experience* a culture of inclusion and sense of belonging that support these policies. Thus, while policies may seemingly support transition into and throughout higher education for marginal groups, the institutional culture can work against this by engendering feelings of alienation and exclusion.

CRITICAL QUESTIONS

+ How can institutions engender a sense of belonging so that students do not develop mental ill-health?

+ How can institutions support new students to adapt to new approaches to learning, teaching and assessment so that stress and anxiety are reduced?

TRANSITION AS INDUCTION

Researchers who have focused on transition as a process of induction into higher education have increasingly moved away from understanding transition as a single point of entry into the university, to increasingly focusing on the first-year experience (Gayle and Parker, 2014). Researchers who are interested in this phase of transition have emphasised the first year of higher education as a complex and challenging period for students (Krause and Coates, 2008), particularly for students from disadvantaged backgrounds (Kift, 2009; Kift and Nelson, 2005; Scanlon et al, 2007). The process of induction requires students

to adjust to the university culture more generally and discipline specific expectations (Beasley and Pearson, 1999). The literature uses
metaphors such as *journey* and *pathway* (Furlong, 2009; Pallas, 2003;
Edvardsson Stiwne and Jungert, 2010) to describe progression through
several phases (Gale and Parker, 2014; Gill et al, 2011).

Many induction programmes in higher education take a holistic
approach by focusing on both curricula induction and co-curricular
induction. This is not surprising given that both academic performance and social integrations are strong predictors of student attrition
(Hillman, 2005). However, Quinn (2010) has argued that the problem
with a focus on transition as induction is that '*the terms of the transition
are set by others*' (p 119). Thus, the process of transition is managed by
institutions that carefully induct students into the values, language and
knowledge which are regarded as institutionally legitimate (Thomas,
2002). Consequently, a successful transition requires students to navigate institutional systems and subscribe to the dominant institutional
culture and values. The limitation of this perspective on transition is
that students do not arrive at institutions as 'empty vessels'. They
arrive with personal values, language, knowledge and interests that
they may need to negotiate to align with the dominant values of the
institution.

CRITICAL QUESTIONS

+ How can institutions empower students by providing them with
  opportunities to co-construct their curriculum and assessments?

+ What impact might this have on their mental health?

TRANSITION AS DEVELOPMENT

Literature that emphasises transition as a process of development
focuses on '*a shift from one identity to another*' (Ecclestone et al, 2010,
p 6) rather than transition as a culmination of experiences. Within the
context of higher education, students develop their identity as a university student. However, university is also a transitional stage (Gale and
Parker, 2014) which serves as a preparation for the development of a
professional identity. Thus, transition at university is also a process
that includes students' development from one life stage to another
(Gale and Parker, 2014).

Researchers who focus on transition as development tend to adopt a perspective from developmental psychology that emphasises the discontinuous nature of the process of development (Werner, 1957). Thus, development is 'stilted' rather than 'smooth' and theorists adopting this position believe that development happens in 'stages' rather than in 'periods' (Gale and Parker, 2014). This is an oppositional perspective to that adopted by theorists who focus on transition as induction. Researchers who adopt a developmental perspective on transition conceptualise transition as a *trajectory* rather a linear pathway to signal a series of cumulative and non-reversible changes (Baron et al, 1999) that shape the development of a student's identity. This trajectory is determined by the individual rather than a predetermined pathway that is mapped out by a social system (Pallas, 2003) and development does not take place at set times.

The two approaches to transition have implications for managing student transitions into and throughout higher education. An emphasis on transition as a process of induction requires students to navigate relatively fixed structures and systems during their first year, while the university 'drip-feeds' specific information to students at specific times so that information is provided '*just in time*' (Gale and Parker, 2014, p 738). An emphasis on transition as a process of development focuses on developing students' identities through processes such as peer mentoring, work-based learning and championing the trajectories of successful alumni (Gale and Parker, 2014). Both perspectives on transition emphasise that the first year of university can be challenging for students. Inductionists emphasise the challenges of new social situations, moving away from home, forming new friendships, financial stress and adapting to studying in higher education as particular situational difficulties that students experience (Hultberg et al, 2009). Conversely, developmentalists emphasise transition as a time of identity reshaping as students' existing views of 'self' and one's place in the world are challenged (Krause and Coates, 2008, p 500). This is particularly evident when students enter universities with practices, traditions and values that are alien to them. For students from disadvantaged areas, this can result in culture shock as students may experience a mismatch between their previous experiences and their new life as a university student.

Differing psychological traditions underpin each of these approaches to transition. If transition is conceptualised as a process of induction, an organisational psychology perspective is most likely to be adopted by researchers. In adopting this psychological perspective, the 'problem' of transition is best addressed through an institutional response. In this model, students are led along a pathway to reach predefined goals (Quinn, 2010). However, researchers who conceptualise transition as development tend to adopt a developmental and social psychology perspective. Rather than necessitating an institutional response to transition, this perspective emphasises the role of individuals and groups in shaping identity and sparking intellectual curiosity (Jamelske, 2009).

CRITICAL QUESTIONS

+ What are the advantages and disadvantages of developing an institutional response to student transition?

+ What are the disadvantages?

TRANSITION AS BECOMING

The concept of transition as a process of becoming (Gale and Parker, 2014) is informed by critical sociology and critical cultural studies. Researchers who conceptualise transition as a process of *becoming* reject the perspective that transitions take place during moments of crisis between relatively stable life experiences (Gale and Parker, 2014). They emphasise that transitions must be negotiated daily and not always in moments of crisis (Ecclestone et al, 2010). 'Becoming' as a concept rejects the notion of moving from one identity to another and embraces multiplicities of self, identity and life choices as well as heterogeneity. These researchers view transition as an everyday occurrence rather than something that is linear and sequential. They reject the metaphor of a pathway to describe the journey of moving on from transition to another. Instead, they embrace the idea that multiple transitions take place every day and that these must be continually negotiated. Analyses of synchronic transitions (Bransford et al, 2006) – transitions between different contexts and *within* the same time frame – are largely absent in the academic literature (Gale and Parker, 2014) and it is these transitions that reflect students' lived experiences at university. Students inhabit multiple physical, cultural, social and psychological domains and they move between several of these domains every day. These transitions between domains are synchronous and do not occur in phases. These transitions are not linear or sequential. Students must learn to negotiate these multiple transitions on a daily basis.

CRITICAL QUESTIONS

+ How might institutions support students to develop an identity as a student and/or researcher?

+ How might institutions support students to develop a professional identity?

+ What other identities might also be developed or developing while students are studying in higher education?

+ How might these multiple identities cause tensions for students?

+ What impact might this have on their mental health?

SUPPORTING STUDENT TRANSITIONS BEYOND THE FIRST YEAR

When students start the second year of their higher education studies you will need to support them in managing the transition from one level of study to the next. At this stage, you will expect them to demonstrate increased independence in managing their own time and their own learning. Students may become anxious or stressed at transferring to a different level of study. You can alleviate this anxiety by meeting with students prior to the transition. In this meeting you will be able to help them to understand:

+ the curriculum content that they will learn over the duration of the year;

+ the assessment tasks that they will be required to complete;

+ the learning outcomes;

+ deadline dates for assessments to support them in managing their time;

+ how their learning will build on their first-year experience;

+ the interrelationship between different elements of the second-year programme.

In the second year of higher education study it is not uncommon for students to demonstrate signs of mental ill-health including stress, anxiety and depression. This is the time when they begin to realise that the 'end goal' of completing their studies is still a long way off. It is also a critical time because students' grades may suddenly start to be more significant for them, particularly if their grades at this level of study start to contribute to their final degree classification. It is also a time when the excitement of higher education may have started to decline for a variety of reasons. Students may have accumulated significant debt by this point in their student journey. They may find their academic work stressful and challenging and they may have to undertake paid work to supplement their finances. The role of the personal tutor is vital to ensure that students are coping well with these increased challenges as they progress to the intermediate stages of their studies. Personal tutors should be aware of a range of warning signs that might indicate that a student is experiencing mental ill-health. These include:

+ persistent absence without authorisation;

+ non-submission of assessed work;

+ a profile of declining academic achievement;

+ withdrawal from social connections;

+ tiredness/lethargy.

Personal tutors play a critical role in supporting students' personal development and making referrals to student support services, usually with the consent of students. Some students prefer to talk to their course leaders or lecturers rather than staff they may not have not met before in student support services. While most lecturers will do their best to support students with personal problems, they are not trained counsellors and they are not qualified to provide financial or disability advice. Personal tutors need to know when a referral needs to be made and when it is appropriate for them to offer advice.

Research highlights that personal tutors need to demonstrate the following attributes:

+ empathy (Ross et al, 2014);

+ friendliness (Bassett et al, 2014);

+ being approachable (Stephen et al, 2008);

+ being non-judgmental (Gubby and McNab, 2013; Wootton, 2013);

+ being genuinely interested in the students (Ross et al, 2014);

+ being caring towards others (Ross et al, 2014);

+ being good listeners (Gubby and McNab, 2013);

+ trustfulness (Dobinson-Harrington, 2006);

+ supportiveness (Stephen et al, 2008);

+ helpfulness.

(cited in Ghenghesh, 2018)

CRITICAL QUESTIONS

+ How can personal tutors negotiate the boundaries of their role with students?

+ Do you think that sessions with personal tutors should be timetabled and made mandatory?

+ Should all academic staff be personal tutors? Explain your answer.

CASE STUDY

One department in a university developed a proactive response to student support. All support staff in the department completed mental health first aid training and some completed a short course in supporting students with mental ill-health. Some staff also completed training in student finance and disability support. Students knew the support staff in the department because they also carried out a dual role as course administrators. A pastoral hub was developed in the department and a drop-in service was operated. This new system operated as a triage; the first line of support was provided by the pastoral team in the department. Students with more severe mental health, financial and disability needs were referred on to university central support services. This model enabled students to get rapid support from people they knew in the department and it reduced the university waiting list for those needing support from central university support services.

SUPPORTING STUDENT TRANSITIONS INTO THE FINAL YEAR

The final year of higher education is very stressful for students. For many undergraduate courses, the grades that students accumulate in the final year will largely determine the final degree classification. This means that students are often under pressure to perform well in the final year of their studies. This can result in stress. Additionally, students are often anxious at this stage about what they will do next. Some will be planning to undertake postgraduate study, some might be planning to travel, and others will plan to undertake employment. As they start their final year, many of these plans are not concrete and their employment opportunities may depend on the degree classification they are awarded. In addition, students will need to make decisions about where they will be living upon completion of their studies and they may be worried about losing contact with the friends they have met during their studies. All these pressures can result in students experiencing stress, anxiety, depression and other forms of mental ill-health.

You can support students during this stage of their education by running a transition event in the summer term before the final year commences. During this event you can make clear the expectations of the final year of study and you can provide an overview of the course modules and assessments. Additionally, you can set the students some tasks to do over the summer so that they can start preparing for their final year. The personal tutor plays a critical role at this stage of the student journey and students might benefit from more regular meetings so that their academic progress and personal development can be more closely monitored during their final year.

Students may be required to undertake a major project, and this can be daunting. Module tutors can prepare students for this task by breaking down the project into a series of smaller steps so that it becomes more manageable for students. Students tend to appreciate being provided with exemplar assignments from past cohorts and mini-deadlines so that they can manage their time and stay on track.

SUPPORTING STUDENT TRANSITIONS INTO PROFESSIONAL PLACEMENTS

While prioritising student satisfaction and responding to the demands of industry, many universities organise work-based learning experiences and professional placements. These develop students' employability skills and provide an opportunity for students to engage with and experience professional contexts (Lemanski et al, 2011). Although often sharing the same objective, approaches to work-based learning and professional placements can vary significantly:

+ summer placements may be offered on an unpaid or paid basis either between years of study or immediately after a student's graduation;

+ industrial placements, usually lasting one year and on a paid basis, are typically offered as part of a student's formal study and may contribute towards the assessment of the qualification;

+ work shadowing placements, often unpaid, may be offered to provide students with a regular and often ongoing opportunity to shadow a member of staff within a professional context, either internally or externally;

+ research placements, often unpaid, may be offered internally and provide students with the opportunity to work alongside university staff in a laboratory or research setting;

+ insight and experience placements, often unpaid, may be used to provide students with an introduction to an area or field to support those considering career and employability pathways.

Despite varying in duration, format and structure, students' exposure to these often new and challenging contexts can contribute to feelings of stress and anxiety.

Universities and tutors play a vital role in supporting students' transitions into professional placements and, in doing so, can alleviate anxieties often contributing to students' mental ill-health.

By embedding opportunities to develop professional skills, through current taught modules, the introduction of focused professional practice modules or recommending workshops offered by the student union, you can equip students with transferable skills to support placement transition:

+ management and leadership skills;

+ communication, consultation and negotiation skills;

+ problem-solving skills;

+ public speaking and presentation skills.

Through developing these skills and exploring their relevance and value, you can increase students' confidence to approach placement opportunities and in doing so reduce the anxieties facing students during this transition.

Developing students' communication, consultation and negotiation skills can provide long-term benefits. These skills provide students with the foundational knowledge required to underpin and support the establishment of professional relationships within a placement context. Establishing these relationships reduces students' anxieties and can support successful academic and professional outcomes.

In cases where these professional relationships break down during placements, students can be left to address and overcome feelings of isolation, failure and depression. As a university tutor, you play a vital role in supporting students whose relationships with work-based mentors may have deteriorated, with negative implications for student mental health.

Tutors as facilitators and remediators can provide students with the advice and support required for them to navigate and negotiate the poor professional relationships affecting their confidence, well-being and mental health. Encouraging students to draw links between practice-based learning and theory is beneficial for students' development. This allows them to recognise the value in their placement experience while simultaneously working alongside university tutors to overcome poor relationships within the placement.

By guiding students to self-reflect on their placement experiences and any feedback offered, you can encourage students to consider their own strengths and those of the placement. Through encouraging self-reflection, the impact of poor professional relationships can be minimised through ensuring students continue to recognise and value the benefits of professional placement opportunities. In supporting these self-reflections, you can also signpost case studies of students who may have faced similar placement experiences. This ensures students can contextualise their own experiences, which reduces feelings of despair and isolation.

When students undertake work placements as part of their degree, they will be expected to demonstrate a range of professional skills. These include:

+ good time management skills;

+ excellent attendance;

+ excellent punctuality;

+ a professional appearance;

+ respect for colleagues;

+ the ability to reflect on their own development;

+ the ability to follow instructions and advice;

+ interpersonal skills.

Some students will already have developed these skills prior to entering higher education but others may need guidance to support them in transitioning from a student to a professional. The personal tutor can support the development of these skills by talking to students about the expectations of professional contexts. Some universities provide all first-year students with sessions on employability to support them in developing these skills and module tutors can embed employability skills into course content and assessment tasks. If students are not supported in developing these skills, they might experience challenges in professional placements that could result in them developing mental ill-health.

CRITICAL QUESTIONS

+ What other skills do students to develop need in professional contexts?

+ In what ways might employability skills be embedded into module content?

CASE STUDY

One small university developed a university-wide approach to pre-paring students for professional placements during the first year of undergraduate study. The central placement team organised a week of work-based learning activities in university prior to all students undertaking a professional placement. The menu of activities included keynote lectures by industry professionals, role-play activities to practise addressing professional challenges, in-tray exercises to develop time management, and problem-based learning. This range of activities ensured that students were fully prepared for their first placements.

SUPPORTING STUDENT TRANSITIONS OUT OF HIGHER EDUCATION

Leaving higher education can be daunting for students, particularly for those students who do not know what they want to do next. Personal tutors can provide advice on routes into postgraduate study and they can support students with job applications. Role-play interviews are also a useful strategy for preparing students for job interviews.

By planning and promoting careers fairs, universities can provide opportunities for students to meet employers and network with recruiters. Through allowing students to build and develop their understanding of the employment process, career fairs can provide information and guidance that informs students' decisions as they prepare to leave higher education.

- 95 per cent of students have reported post-university depression.
- 87 per cent of students interviewed feel there should be more exposure of post-university depression to highlight the issues.

(www.independent.co.uk/student/student-life/health/graduate-blues-why-we-need-to-talk-about-post-university-depression-8729522.html)

Research suggests that one of the reasons that some students do not have a positive experience of higher education when they start their university courses is because there is often a 'gap' between their expectations and their initial experiences or reality (Leese, 2010; Parkinson and Forrester, 2004).

Strategies to support student transition include the establishment of friendship and peer support networks to mitigate social isolation (Ribchester et al, 2014), access to tutors (Schreiner et al, 2011) and pre-induction social networking (Ribchester et al, 2014). Studies suggest that students leave their courses due to academic reasons, financial pressures, physical and mental health problems, dissatisfaction with the university, homesickness, location, campus climate and culture and family issues (Cole, 2017; Morrow and Ackermann, 2012). Trautwein and Bosse (2017) found that both academic and social integration are critical for a smooth transition to university and concluded that transition through the first year of university is a multifaceted process that unfolds in stages as the student interacts with institutional, social and academic contexts.

Despite the documented strategies that support transition, Reason (2009) argued that *'we need to stop searching for a silver bullet'* (p 678), because strategies that work on one campus may not necessarily work on another.

 41 per cent of 16 to 24 year-olds felt overwhelmed when facing university transitions.

(www.independent.co.uk/student/istudents/students-and-mental-health-what-to-do-if-you-re-struggling-at-university-a6778576.html)

SUMMARY

This chapter has explored the importance of facilitating smooth transitions throughout higher education study, work-based learning and professional placements. Smooth transitions between these can alleviate anxieties and reduce the mental health difficulties experienced by students. It has highlighted the critical role of tutors in ensuring students are prepared for and supported during professional placements and the impact of the tutor on a student's confidence and mental health. The role of the university in supporting students leaving higher education has been explained and related strategies explored.

CHECKLIST

This chapter has addressed:

✓ the significance of tutor support in ensuring smooth transitions between phases of higher education, professional placements and work-based learning;

✓ the value of tutor support for students whose experiences involve deteriorating relationships in professional placements and work-based learning;

✓ the importance of extending efforts to support transition beyond the final year of a student's study.

FURTHER READING

Neugebauer, J and Evans-Brain, J (2009) *Making the Most of Your Placement*. London: Sage Publications.

✚ CHAPTER 7

SUPPORTING TRANSITIONS OUT OF HIGHER EDUCATION

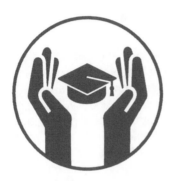

PROFESSIONAL LINKS

This chapter addresses the following:

The Unite Students Insight Report 2016 sets out findings from a major student survey. A key finding was the interconnectedness of student life: students who have a positive experience in one area are much more likely to have a positive experience in other areas. Positive experiences are linked to emotional resilience, positive mental well-being and social integration. The report also addresses employment-related issues for students who are transitioning out of higher education.

CHAPTER OBJECTIVES

After reading this chapter you will understand:

+ the challenges experienced by students in their final year of higher education;

+ the role of academic and professional service teams in addressing these challenges.

INTRODUCTION

The final year of higher education can be particularly challenging for students. At this stage, students may experience significant stress due to increased workloads and the high-stakes nature of assessments in the final year. Many students place significant pressure on themselves because they want to perform academically at a high level. They have invested significant time and financial resources into their studies, and this can result in a desire to get the best grade possible. In addition, students are very aware that the employment market is extremely competitive. To stand a chance of successfully gaining graduate employment, students may feel that they need to academically outperform other students, even though employers often seek a broader range of skills.

In the final year of a degree course, academic pressures are only part of the problem. Students may feel pressured to make decisions about their future careers. While some students will, by this stage, know what they want to do, others may not, and this can result in an additional layer of stress on top of academic pressures. In addition, students may also have to decide where they want to live and work when they have completed their studies. At this stage of the student lifecycle, students may have accumulated significant debt. This may result in them developing mental ill-health, particularly if they have no means to begin repayments. Some students may have to face the prospect of living back at home with their family, following three or four years of relative independence. This may not be an ideal prospect for some students, who may be keen to retain their independence, especially given the fact that they are now young adults.

This chapter addresses these challenges but also considers the implications for academic and student service teams within the institution.

FINAL-YEAR CHALLENGES

For most undergraduate students, the final year of their studies is the most critical year. Their degree classification may largely be dependent upon their performance in the final year and many students will study on courses that have final examinations. Students may place significant pressure on themselves to perform highly and this can result in a range of mental health conditions including stress, anxiety, depression, eating disorders and self-harm. This 'self-pressure' may be the result of students knowing that they have invested significant time and resources into their studies and achieving a good result can help justify this.

During the final year of higher education and during their transition out of higher education, students experience multiple and multidimensional transitions that can detrimentally impact on their mental health. These include:

+ adjusting to the academic demands of the course, including course content and the level they are required to work at;

+ psychological transitions: transitioning from a student identity to a professional identity;

+ geographical transitions: making decisions about where they want to live and work;

+ social transitions: the prospect of losing touch with friends who they have spent significant time with and then adjusting to new friendships.

CRITICAL QUESTIONS

+ How can lecturers prepare students for the academic demands of the final year?

+ What are the implications for the personal tutor in relation to supporting students during the final year?

+ What are the implications for professional service teams?

- Young adults aged 20–24 are less likely than any other age group to record high levels of well-being (life satisfaction, feeling that things done in life are worthwhile, happiness and low anxiety).

- Between 2007 and 2015, the number of student suicides increased by 79 per cent (from 75 to 134).

- Suicide is often linked to the presence of mental health conditions, although victims of suicide may not have accessed mental health services.

- In 2014/15, a significant number of students (1,180) who experienced mental health problems withdrew from university, an increase of 210 per cent compared to 2009/10.

(Thorley, C (2017) *Not by Degrees: Improving Student Mental Health in the UK's Universities*. IPPR)

THE ROLE OF THE PERSONAL TUTOR IN THE FINAL YEAR

Some students may need to spend more time with their personal tutor during the final year, particularly if they are experiencing mental ill-health. The pressure to perform is often not transmitted to students by academic staff but emerges from the students who are usually motivated to do well. Personal tutors, course leaders and lecturers should be vigilant to the signs of mental ill-health in students. These may include:

+ declining attendance;

+ changes in mood and/or behaviour;

+ social isolation, avoiding contact;

+ changes in physical appearance;

+ declining academic performance.

Students' mental health can also be affected by external factors. While they may be coping with the academic demands of the final year of their studies, the balance can easily be tipped by additional factors, which can then result in students feeling that they are unable to cope. These factors could include illness, the death of someone close to them, changes in their family circumstances and community-related factors.

When things go wrong in the lives of students, these factors can result in students then feeling that they cannot cope, and these students may need additional support from their personal tutor and other services in the university.

The problem for personal tutors is that there is ambiguity over the role. Some personal tutors may feel inadequately prepared for addressing pastoral issues and this highlights the need for a clear, comprehensive professional development programme for everyone holding this role. Some personal tutors may feel that there should be a clear separation between pastoral and academic support, while others may feel that the two are interrelated. Clearly, if students are experiencing mental ill-health, this will impact on their academic performance. Training for personal tutors is vital so that they are clear when they should address students' needs and when and how they should refer cases on to student services.

Problems also arise when students contact personal tutors out of hours. There needs to be clarity over whose role it is to provide support to students in the evenings and weekends and this should be stated within institutional policies and explicitly communicated to students. The boundaries of the role should be made clear to students from the start.

Given the fact that personal tutors are likely to provide students with mental health advice, it seems reasonable to suggest that the institution should create opportunities and spaces for tutors to come together to share practice and concerns. This would provide a valuable opportunity to support personal tutors in their roles. Additionally, given the fact that personal tutors may be giving advice to students in relation to their mental health, institutions should consider providing them with regular, impartial supervision so that they are provided with frequent opportunities to discuss their 'cases' anonymously. The supervisor plays an important role in providing reassurance to the personal tutor that they have made the right decision or suggesting alternative approaches. Professional supervision is common in the health professions and social care but not in education. Given the increased expectations on education staff to address students' mental health needs, there is a clear need to develop this practice in education settings.

Personal tutors may feel detached from professional service teams in the university. There is a clear need to improve communication between professional service teams and academics and one way of addressing this is through joint training. There is also a need to develop a shared language between different services so that good communication is facilitated. Leaders and managers should help staff to understand other people's roles and responsibilities so that there is clarity within the institution in relation to lines of responsibility and accountability.

CRITICAL QUESTIONS

+ What are the implications for personal tutors if they provide the 'wrong' advice to students in relation to their mental health?

+ How might personal tutors help students to plan, organise and manage their workload?

+ When should personal tutors refer students to other services?

THE ROLE OF MENTAL HEALTH SUPPORT TEAMS

Most institutions operate a suite of mental health services for students, including access to counselling, psychologists, sexual health advice and trained therapists. The student union may also operate separate services for students. Mental health support teams can provide tailored programmes of intervention or treatment to students with mental health needs. These services also play a role in supporting the professional development of academics and other professional services teams who have contact with students in relation to mental health.

Mental health support teams are a critical part of the university infrastructure. They enable students to get the support they need so that they can continue with their studies and they support students to become mentally healthy. However, it is important to note that many services in institutions are over-stretched with too few staff working with large numbers of students. This can result in untimely referrals and therefore students not receiving the support when they need it.

It is critical that academic staff, including personal tutors, course leaders, year leaders, heads of department and lecturing staff know when and how to refer students to mental health services. If you work within the mental health service team, it is crucial that you explicitly state to students what the remit of your role is, what level of support they can expect to receive and the boundaries of your role. Students may also need to know how they can access support outside of working hours and what services may exist within the community.

CRITICAL QUESTIONS

+ What are the benefits of a university counselling service?
+ When is it appropriate to refer students to a counselling service and when might it not be appropriate?
+ What are the differences between the mental health advice that academics can offer, and the support offered by mental health support teams?

THE ROLE OF ACADEMIC SKILLS SERVICES

During the final year, students may experience significant mental ill-health as they adjust to the academic standard needed to successfully pass their course. Academic staff can facilitate a smooth academic transition by leading workshops with students in the summer term immediately prior to the final year. During these workshops you can introduce students to the academic standard, and you can also share with them samples of work from previous students so that they can see the standard that they will be expected to achieve.

Some institutions have established academic skills teams to support students in the development of the skills they need to perform at all levels of academic study. These services are particularly useful to all students in the final year because students can be supported to refine their academic skills so that they can attain at a higher level. These services tend to operate through an appointment booking system. Students who need support to reach a pass standard can access these services as well as highly performing students who want to excel even further. Students working between these two extremes can also benefit through tailored support to help them develop the skills to perform at a higher level. Institutions can market these services by academic skills tutors raising the profile of the service by attending classes at the start of the academic year.

CRITICAL QUESTIONS

+ If numbers of students seeking academic support increase, how can academic skills services become sustainable?

+ The operational model of one-to-one support is costly and time-consuming. What alternative models of academic skills support could exist?

THE ROLE OF CAREERS SERVICES

The university careers service plays a crucial role in supporting students to gain employment, both during their studies and upon completion of their studies. Most careers services offer an appointments service or drop-in service so that students can gain bespoke advice about writing a curriculum vitae, applying for jobs, marketing themselves on social media and specific support with interview preparation. In addition, careers services can also assist students to develop volunteering experiences and internal work experience that will help them to develop a range of skills and improve their confidence. Careers services teams can provide additional support by leading lectures within modules during the final year on careers-related issues. Careers teams can play an important role in reviewing the learning outcomes and skills that are embedded within taught modules to ensure that graduate employment skills are being developed throughout the course of study. Integrating graduate employability skills through the taught curriculum will ensure that students develop the knowledge, skills and confidence they need throughout their course to make them employable.

Research by O'Leary (2016) demonstrated that 90 per cent of 104 graduates from humanities, sciences, engineering and social sciences wanted discipline-specific employability skills to have a greater emphasis in their course. Ninety per cent of graduates emphasised the need to provide greater focus on employability compared to 10 per cent of graduates who preferred to develop subject-specific knowledge, skills and understanding. These findings have implications for careers services to further develop their involvement within taught programmes.

- Most students at UK universities recognise the support and development they receive from their university to prepare them for employment.

- Two-thirds of students feel that their university is preparing them well for employment after graduation. This is made up of 18 per cent who feel 'very well prepared' for employment after graduation and 47 per cent who feel 'somewhat well prepared'.

- A much smaller proportion, 13 per cent, feel their universities prepare them poorly for employment after graduation.

- Students from lower socioeconomic groups are more likely than those from higher socioeconomic groups to feel poorly prepared by their university for employment after graduation.

- About two-thirds of students reported that they would go to a careers service at their university for help applying for jobs (65 per cent), for career skills (65 per cent) and for advice or support about choosing a career (62 per cent).

- Many students are not confident about their future career opportunities. Only one in ten students (9 per cent) feel that it will be very easy to get the job that they want after graduating. Most students are less optimistic with close to two-fifths (36 per cent) feeling that it is going to be a challenge and a further 8 per cent assuming it will be almost impossible to get a job they want when they graduate.

- Students from lower socioeconomic groups are less likely than others to find graduate employment even at 40 months post-graduation.

(Unite Students Insight Report, 2016, www.unitestudents.com/about-us/insightreport/2016-full-report)

CASE STUDY

One department in a university developed an external mentoring scheme to support final-year students in gaining graduate employment. Journalism students were paired with professional journalists, many of whom were alumni of the university. The mentor's role was to specifically support the student to gain graduate employment within the sector. The mentor met with the student at the start of the academic year to develop an agreement about the operational aspects of the scheme including:

+ frequency of meetings;

+ the types of support and experiences that the mentor would provide;

+ boundaries of the role.

Some mentors provided students with industry experience at times when students were not timetabled to attend lectures. All mentors provided specific tailored support on writing a curriculum vitae, developing a professional social media platform so that students could market themselves, applying for jobs and interview preparation. Some mentors developed a suite of industry experiences for their students so that students could make decisions about which aspect of the sector they wanted to work in.

CRITICAL QUESTIONS

+ What are the barriers to graduates seeking employment?

+ The Teaching Excellence Framework holds higher education institutions to account in relation to graduate employment. To what extent is this fair?

+ How might emphasising graduate employment within the Teaching Excellence Framework disadvantage some higher education institutions?

THE ROLE OF DISABILITY SUPPORT SERVICES

Disability support services play a crucial role throughout the student lifecycle in assessing the needs of students with disabilities, developing personalised learning and support plans and ensuring that reasonable adjustments are in place so that students with disabilities have equality of opportunity. While these arrangements may suit the student throughout their studies, the needs of students with disabilities must also be reviewed by the disability services team prior to the commencement of final year study. This supports students whose needs may have changed during their studies and ensures appropriate adjustments are in place to support the student at this critical time in their course.

Research by the Equality Challenge Unit (ECU, 2014) demonstrates that among students with experience of mental ill-health, the main reason given for not talking to other students about their mental health was *'not wanting students to think less of them'*. However, despite this fear, research does suggest that most students are sympathetic to those who experience mental illness (Aronin and Smith, 2016). Research demonstrates that students may also opt not to disclose their condition if they believe they are likely to be subjected to institutional stigma or prejudice from staff. Students who do not disclose mental ill-health fear that they will receive *'unfair treatment'* as a result (ECU, 2014). In addition, students perceive disclosure as limiting future opportunities.

CASE STUDY

Students studying a programme of initial teacher training were provided with a bespoke package of support to enable them to thrive in their first year of teaching. This support included the following:

+ the development of a charter that explicitly outlined the role of the university in supporting students beyond graduation;

+ a menu of support opportunities during the first year of employment;

+ support in applying for teaching posts and interview preparation that extended beyond graduation;

+ an autumn term 'drop in' session so that graduates could return to the university to meet with lecturers and former students;

+ a conference in the spring term during the first year of employment, which included influential keynote lectures;

+ a telephone hotline for graduates who needed support during the first year of employment;

+ the development of a social media site so that lecturers and students could keep in touch;

+ access to an online platform so that graduates could gain access to the latest teaching resources.

CRITICAL QUESTIONS

+ How might this model be applied to other courses?
+ Why do higher education institutions play an important role in supporting students and graduates 'from the cradle to the grave'?

SUMMARY

This chapter has outlined some of the challenges that students might experience during their final year. It has explored the implications of these for the personal tutor and disability and careers services within the university. Strategies to support students throughout their final-year studies have been identified and case study examples have been used to illuminate best practice.

CHECKLIST

This chapter has addressed:

✓ the need for personal tutors to know when to refer students to mental health services;

✓ the necessity for employability skills to be embedded through the curriculum;

✓ the role that external mentors can play in supporting graduate employability skills;

✓ the importance of developing clear communication between academic staff and staff in professional service teams.

FURTHER READING

Matheson, R (2018) *Transition In, Through and Out of Higher Education*. London: Routledge.

CHAPTER 8

SUPPORTING THE MENTAL HEALTH NEEDS OF POSTGRADUATE STUDENTS

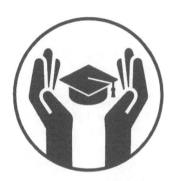

PROFESSIONAL LINKS

This chapter addresses the following:

A research project undertaken on behalf of the Higher Education Funding Council for England (HEFCE) explored the well-being and mental health of postgraduate research students (Metcalfe et al, 2018).

CHAPTER OBJECTIVES

After reading this chapter you will understand:

+ the challenges experienced by postgraduate research students and the impact of these on their mental health;

+ the implications for research supervisors who work with postgraduate students.

INTRODUCTION

Studying at postgraduate level can be both exciting and daunting at the same time. Students are usually enthusiastic about their research topic and keen to develop new skills and knowledge. At the same time, studying at this level is very different to undergraduate study. Postgraduate research students are usually expected to determine their own research focus, unless they have secured a scholarship to conduct a specific piece of research. They will be expected to work largely independently and manage their own time. They will be expected to develop their own research proposal and plan of implementation. Students working at this level usually have greater knowledge of their topic than their supervisors, who may be experts in the research process, but they will not necessarily have conducted the same research that their students are conducting.

Studying at postgraduate level can be a lonely experience. There may be no taught sessions and all teaching may be based on a model of supervision. Students may have limited opportunities to interact with other research students and some students will be studying at distance and supervisions may be conducted using video conferencing. Some students may start to feel isolated and this can result in mental ill-health.

This chapter introduces you to some of these challenges and considers others too. It focuses on the implications for research supervisors who are in a critical position to impact on students' mental health.

INDUCTING STUDENTS INTO POSTGRADUATE STUDY

Many students starting postgraduate research courses develop 'imposter syndrome'. They often cannot believe that they have been accepted to study at a high level and they may initially lack confidence in their own abilities and demonstrate signs of anxiety. These are typical feelings at an early stage, and it is important to acknowledge how students are feeling and to reassure them that they will gradually start to feel more confident and less anxious as their studies progress.

Most universities run an induction event to postgraduate study, even if students are studying via distance learning. It is important to encourage student attendance at an induction event because this is where you can acknowledge how students are feeling, provide students with guidance on the roles and responsibilities of both students and supervisors, and provide opportunities for students to listen to presentations by current and past postgraduate students. These events also provide valuable opportunities to develop a community of research students, develop a sense of belonging and connectedness to the institution and enable students to begin to form academic and social connections and networks. Each of these can impact positively on students' mental health.

If attendance at a face-to-face induction is not possible, research supervisors should aim to provide an induction experience using the virtual learning platform. Discussion boards can be useful to enable students to introduce themselves to others and to facilitate student and staff collaboration. A live synchronous session using video conferencing software is also a very effective strategy for enabling students and staff to meet virtually.

Research programmes now vary significantly in design and assessment. Some, particularly professional doctorates, may include taught elements with assessment tasks that students are required to complete. Some programmes may include no taught elements. Some research programmes are assessed through submission of a thesis. Others may be assessed through submission of a product or a combination of a thesis and a product. Others may be assessed through an element of practice-based work within a professional context, supported by a written commentary. Some students may be undertaking doctorates through publication of assessed work in books, chapters or academic journals. Students should have researched the programme they have selected to ensure that it meets their own requirements.

SETTING BOUNDARIES IN THE STUDENT–SUPERVISOR RELATIONSHIP

A significant and critical element of postgraduate study is supervision. Models of supervision vary between institutions. In some institutions, students are supervised by a research team rather than a single supervisor. They may be allocated a main supervisor, but they may also be allocated a second or even third supervisor. In other institutions, students may only be attached to one supervisor.

If you are working as part of a research supervision team, it is important that you establish some protocols that will frame how you will work together to provide the best experience for the student. You will need to negotiate:

+ the roles and responsibilities of each person in the research team;

+ the frequency of supervisions, considering institutional policies;

+ whether you will conduct joint supervisions or separate supervisions;

+ whether one person will provide the student with feedback on their work or whether all members of the team will review work and provide feedback;

+ what can reasonably be expected of students prior to attending a supervision;

+ what aspects of the research process different people in the research team will take responsibility for.

In an ideal world, supervisors will have been assigned a specific student based on their expertise of the research topic or the methodological approach that will underpin the study. However, this may not always be the case. It is important to be very explicit with the student about what each person can contribute to the research process so that the student understands the roles and responsibilities of each person in the research team.

Once you have set protocols to guide how you will work as a research team, you will need to establish professional boundaries with research students. While it may seem strange to use this term, especially given that some research students may also be your academic colleagues, nevertheless it is important to be very clear about your expectations from the outset so that there is no ambiguity. Establishing boundaries with the student may include being very explicit about the following:

+ the frequency of supervisions;

+ their responsibilities in relation to preparing for supervision;

+ their responsibilities to act on feedback following supervision sessions;

+ the amount of output they are expected to produce by specific milestones;

+ how much work you will review and expected timescales for feedback;

+ when you can be contacted;

+ how frequently can you be contacted;

+ how you should be contacted (for example, email, telephone, video conferencing, via social media);

+ what you and other members of the research team can contribute to the project;

+ times during the year when you are not available due to holidays or international work;

+ how your role will change as students move through a project.

CRITICAL QUESTIONS

+ Why is it important to establish these boundaries with students?

+ Are there any other boundaries that have not been identified above that you think need to be set?

You should be very clear with students in relation to how you expect them to prepare for supervisory sessions. Some supervisors expect students to send them some work to review in advance of a supervision session. This is an effective strategy because it creates a focus for the supervision. However, you may need to explicitly state to students that you expect them to send you the work in a reasonable timescale in advance of the meeting.

NEGOTIATING PROFESSIONAL RELATIONSHIPS WITH STUDENTS

So much depends on the quality of the student–supervisor relationship for students who are studying on postgraduate research programmes. The supervision process is the primary tool that will shape students' thinking. For students studying on PhD programmes, it is likely to be the only teaching that students will receive. It is therefore crucial that students feel comfortable with their supervisor.

A good supervisor empowers students in various ways. These might include:

+ developing students' self-concept and self-esteem so that they believe that they can succeed;

+ fostering motivation;

+ showing a genuine interest in students' research projects;

+ challenging students intellectually;

+ supporting the student at times when they will inevitably feel overwhelmed;

+ asking questions that promote reflection;

+ initiating contact with students who may be avoiding contact with their supervisor or those who are not making adequate progress;

+ preparing their students for institutional milestones such as formal progress meetings;

+ preparing their students for the final assessment.

It is important for supervisors to demonstrate empathy towards their students. Undertaking a research degree is no mean feat and there are likely to be times when students feel overwhelmed to the point that they may want to withdraw. You can support them through these points by explaining that their feelings are typical and that it is usual to experience feelings of being in the middle of 'fog' and to not know where one is heading. Spending time listening to your students' perspectives is time that is well-invested.

It is also important for supervisors to recognise that many students who study on postgraduate research degrees at master's or doctoral level are increasingly starting these programmes alongside other commitments in their lives, particularly if they have opted to study them while they are in full-time employment. Many students are embarking on research programmes at a stage when they are mid-career. They may have family commitments, including parenting responsibilities or caring commitments to older relatives. They may have a demanding full-time professional job. They may have financial commitments such as mortgages that have to be paid regularly. Sometimes, the research degree is further down their list of priorities than they would ideally want, and this can impact on timely completion of the programme. Some students may need to suspend their studies for a period of time, particularly if their external priorities change or become overwhelming. Having a supervisor who understands the pressures that students are experiencing makes all the difference and can determine whether students complete their programmes successfully.

CASE STUDY

One university developed a mentoring scheme for all students on doctoral programmes. Each student was provided with access to a confidential mentor who was not involved in supervising the student. The supervisor was not allowed to know the identity of the mentor. The mentors were selected from across the university and allocated to students who were based in a different faculty. The role of the mentor was to provide students with advice about a range of aspects of the doctoral journey including independent advice on the supervisory relationship. In cases where students had expressed concerns about the supervisory relationship, mentors informed the lead for doctoral programmes in the faculty and the issues were investigated.

Wellington and Sikes (2006) found that students studying on professional doctorate programmes experienced several personal challenges during their studies. These included the breakdown of personal relationships due to doctorate commitments and feelings of guilt after spending less time with elderly relatives. In some cases, relationships with family members became strained due to the pressures of studying on the programme.

BEING A CRITICAL FRIEND

Good supervisors recognise that they must act as a critical friend to their students. You may not be an expert in the student's choice of topic but, nevertheless, you recognise what a good research study looks like and you will have a strong understanding of the research process. You may have also been involved in externally examining submissions for research degrees and your insight from these experiences will be invaluable.

Many students who embark on research degrees believe that their knowledge of the area of study is the most critical thing. While it is important for students to demonstrate mastery of the topic, it is equally important that they can demonstrate mastery of the research design. As a supervisor, you play an important role in both supporting and encouraging your students, but also in asking critical questions that will challenge them intellectually. It is important to strike a balance between being overly and unnecessarily critical and being too positive and too supportive. Many students studying research degrees will be required to undertake a final oral assessment known as a viva voce. This provides the student with an opportunity to defend their work. Asking challenging questions throughout the process will prepare your students well for this final assessment and will improve the overall quality of their work.

However, when relationships between students and supervisors break down this can have a significant and detrimental impact on the students. Studying for a research degree can be an isolating and stressful experience. If students feel that their supervisor does not like them and is overly critical of their work, and if they feel that they may not complete the programme successfully, this can result in disengagement and demotivation. As a supervisor you hold a significant amount of power over your student. However, this power should be used wisely, and it should never be abused. While you have a vested interest in your students successfully completing their programmes, it is worth bearing in mind that it is not your study. Students retain overall ownership of their work and therefore you should try to avoid 'over-shaping' the study to the extent that students end up taking a completely different path to the one they intended. It is also worth bearing in mind that your students may have financially invested into their programmes and therefore you have a responsibility to meet your obligations as a supervisor. This also applies to students who have secured scholarships.

Awareness of the factors contributing to the mental ill-health of undergraduate students has been well documented by many. Despite this, research focusing on the mental health of postgraduate students remains limited. A report undertaken by Vitae on behalf of the former Higher Education Funding Council for England (HEFCE) researched the risk factors impacting the mental health of postgraduate research students. Postgraduate research students and university staff from ten institutions were interviewed and the influences on the well-being and mental health of these students were explored. In their report, Metcalfe et al (2018) found that the following factors influenced the well-being and mental health of postgraduate research students:

+ expectations of high achievement triggering imposter syndrome;

+ difficulties with supervisory relationships;

+ reluctance to discuss well-being issues and fearing the impact of initiating these conversations;

+ for international students, new culture, finance and visa adjustments;

+ reduced accessibility of existing friends and family support networks.

Responding to these pressures, higher education institutions continue to prioritise their offer in terms of student support services and procedures for identifying and addressing students' mental ill-health. The report's conclusion finds that the mental health and well-being of postgraduate research students can only be supported in cases where institutions develop and embed systemic culture changes and a strategic commitment to promoting positive mental health.

ASSESSING STUDENTS' WORK

It is usual practice for postgraduate research students to send drafts of their work to their supervisors for formative feedback. On many postgraduate research programmes, you may not have responsibility for assessing the final submission and the final assessment may be completed by internal and external examiners. However, your formative feedback is crucial in ensuring that students are working at the relevant academic standard and therefore you should see yourself as a critical friend. Your role is to draw the student's attention to what is good about their work and to make suggestions for improvement.

How you frame your feedback is crucial. Students, especially at the start of a research programme, often lack confidence. Overly critical feedback can impact detrimentally on the student's self-belief and confidence and may even result in some students withdrawing from their programme. It is important to start by identifying the strengths of the work before you identify areas for development. It is also essential to support your comments with examples so that students understand exactly what they need to do to ensure that the work reaches the correct academic standard.

You should be aware of how your comments on a piece of work can impact on how the student feels. When you are writing feedback, you should be sensitive to how your comments might be interpreted. Comments should relate to the student's work and should not be personal. One example of this is the following comment: '*It is a pity that you did not attend your supervision session because, had you done so, your work would have been much better.*' This comment is personal because it is a criticism of the student. It is also ineffective as a piece of feedback because it does not show why the work does not meet the required standards and the student has not been given advice about what they need to do to improve.

CRITICAL QUESTIONS

+ Can you give an example of an effective feedback comment?
+ Should supervisors be more critical in their feedback so that students can reach a higher standard?

BUILDING A RESEARCH COMMUNITY

Studying for a research degree can be a particularly isolating experience if students are not provided with opportunities to network and collaborate with other students. Supervisors should provide opportunities to meet and share their work, even if this is done virtually. Collaborative conferencing software is effective for conducting virtual meetings. If students feel isolated during their research journey then there is a risk that they will experience mental ill-health.

WORKING WITH INTERNATIONAL STUDENTS

Many international students come to the United Kingdom to study research degrees. They may be anxious about their ability to write in clear English and they may be worried about family members in their home country. They need to quickly adapt to a new country and to a new community. They also need to adapt to the education system, which may be very different to the system they are used to.

As the supervisor, you can help them to feel more included by:

+ building informal social communities of international students who meet regularly as a group and participate in a range of extra-curricular activities, such as visiting places of interest;

+ developing cultural sensitivity – learn as much as you can about their culture, including cultural norms and values, and integrate this cultural knowledge into supervisions;

+ including international students in university research events, such as student-led conferences and lectures;

+ explaining at the start the format of the feedback that you will provide and that critical commentary on their work is not a personal attack;

+ being aware that is not culturally acceptable for some students to be in a room alone with a supervisor and therefore you might need to conduct supervisions in shared open spaces, such as the library.

PREPARING STUDENTS FOR EXAMINATION

Most research degrees are assessed through a viva voce examination. Understandably students can become nervous about this because it is a formal event and much rides on completing it successfully. You can support your students to prepare for this by providing them with examples of the types of questions that they might be asked and discussing possible responses with them. Sometimes this is referred to as a 'mock viva'.

It is equally important to prepare your students with other aspects of the viva, including:

+ what to wear (formal or informal dress);

+ how to annotate their thesis;

+ body posture;

+ body language;

+ how to respond to a critical line of questioning;

+ the importance of eye contact and enthusiasm.

While the viva is an assessment of the academic work, there is an element of performance and your students will need to be prepared to project themselves with passion and confidence about their research.

CRITICAL QUESTIONS

+ How might a mock viva affect the supervisory relationship?

+ How might a mock viva impact on students' mental health?

+ How might supervisor presence within the viva influence a student's experiences?

🌑 0.9 per cent of postgraduate students declared mental ill-health, while 3.3 per cent of this population reported experiencing mental ill-health.

🌑 The General Health Questionnaire (GHQ) identified that 32 per cent of the postgraduate researcher community are at risk of having or developing a psychiatric disorder, such as depression.

(Metcalfe et al, 2018)

CASE STUDY

One university developed a mandatory training course that all research supervisors were required to undertake. The course addressed aspects such as managing the student–supervisor relationship, models of support and the factors that can cause mental ill-health in students. Supervisors were taught to recognise the signs of mental ill-health in their research students. They were provided with guidance about how to support students experiencing mental ill-health and when and how to refer students, with their consent, to mental health services in the university.

- 58 per cent of male postgraduate researcher students reported that they had never consulted their peers about their mental health, compared with 45 per cent of female students.

- 29 per cent of male postgraduate research students stated that they had not consulted their family and friends about their mental health, compared with 15 per cent of female students.

(Metcalfe et al, 2018)

SUMMARY

This chapter has explored many of the challenges facing postgraduate students as they move through their study. These typically include students developing feelings of anxiousness, isolation and loneliness. The factors contributing to these feelings have been highlighted and the role of supervisors in supporting students' mental health has been discussed. The role of a supervisor often includes providing formative feedback, preparing students for assessment, providing opportunities for students to network and inducting students to their postgraduate study. Through offering students these experiences, supervisors can play a crucial role in alleviating students' anxieties and supporting their positive mental health and academic success.

CHECKLIST

This chapter has addressed:

✓ the challenges facing postgraduate students and the impact of these on mental health and well-being;

✓ the importance of supervisory relationships in supporting and promoting students' positive mental health;

✓ the practical strategies available to supervisors to alleviate students' anxieties and address the factors contributing to mental ill-health.

FURTHER READING

McMaster, C, Murphy, C, Cronshaw, S and McMaster, N (2016) *Postgraduate Study in the UK: Surviving and Succeeding*. London: Libri Publishing.

✚ CONCLUSION

As stated at the start of this book, student mental health in higher education is the concern of everyone who works in the institution.

We have emphasised the need for an institution-wide approach to mental health that eradicates stigma. We have argued that supporting students' mental health extends beyond the support that is provided to students who demonstrate signs of mental ill-health. The institution-wide approach demonstrates a commitment enabling all students and staff to be mentally healthy while studying or working at the university.

It is a concern that declining student mental ill-health appears to be on the increase. There is insufficient research on the causes of this at present to establish the reasons for this 'crisis'. We suspect that the reasons are complex and multifaceted. However, while media attention is given to undergraduate students, we have emphasised the need for universities to pay more attention to the mental health of postgraduate students, particularly those who are studying research degrees. We have also emphasised the need for universities to give greater attention to the mental health of students following distance-learning courses who may never need to attend the physical campus. These groups of students are often overlooked.

We have argued that universities need to give greater attention to supporting students' mental health and that this should be a strategic institutional priority. We have also argued that universities should report to governing bodies regularly on student mental health and we have highlighted the need for staff training in mental health.

Many young people develop mental ill-health by the age of 14 and these problems can continue into adulthood. Schools and colleges are now giving increased attention to supporting the mental health of children and young people and we are hopeful that this will pay dividends long-term. We have emphasised the need for educational institutions to monitor the impact of their mental health provision and to adjust provision in cases where interventions are deemed to be less effective. We have also emphasised the need to involve students in all discussions about the support they require to enable them to complete their studies successfully.

+REFERENCES

Aronin, S and Smith, M (2016)
One in Four Students Suffer from Mental Health Problems. YouGov, 9 August 2016. [online] Available at: https://yougov.co.uk/topics/lifestyle/articles-reports/2016/08/09/quarter-britains-students-are-afflicted-mental-hea (accessed 9 January 2019).

Askham, P (2008)
Context and Identity: Exploring Adult Learners' Experiences of Higher Education. *Journal of Further and Higher Education*, 32(1): 85–97.

Baron, S, Riddell, S and Wilson, A (1999)
The Secret of Eternal Youth: Identity, Risk and Learning Difficulties. *British Journal of Sociology of Education*, 20(4): 483–99.

Bassett, J, Gallagher, E and Price, L (2014)
Personal Tutors' Responses to a Structured System of Personal Development Planning: A Focus on 'Feedback'. *Journal for Education in the Built Environment*, 9(1): 22–34.

Bauman, Z (2001)
The Individualized Society. Cambridge: Polity Press.

Beasley, C J and Pearson, C A L (1999)
Facilitating the Learning of Transitional Students: Strategies for Success for All Students. *Higher Education Research and Development*, 18(3): 303–21.

Belyakov, A, Cremonini, L, Mfusi, M X and Rippner, J (2009)
The Effect of Transitions on Access to Higher Education. Washington, DC: Institute for Higher Education Policy.

Bonassi, T and Wolter, S C (2002)
Measuring the Success of Transition: The Results of a Pre-Study in Switzerland. *Education and Training*, 44(4–5): 199–207.

Bransford, J, Stevens, R, Schwartz, D, Meltzoff, A, Pea, R, Roschelle, J, Vye, N, et al (2006)
Learning Theories and Education: Toward a Decade of Synergy. In Alexander, P and Winne, P (eds) *Handbook of Educational Psychology* (pp 209–44). Mahwah, NJ: Erlbaum.

Briggs, A, Clark, J and Hall, I (2012)
Building Bridges: Understanding Student Transition to University. *Journal of Quality in Higher Education*, 18(1): 3–21.

Browne, K (2008)
Imagining Cities, Living the Other: Between the Gay Urban Idyll and Rural Lesbian Lives. *The Open Geography Journal International*, 1: 25–32.

Burnett, L (2007)
Juggling First Year Student Experiences and Institutional Changes: An Australian Experience. Paper presented at the 20th International Conference on First Year Experience, July, in Hawaii, USA. [online] Available at: https://research-repository.griffith.edu.au/bitstream/handle/10072/32622/51648_1.pdf (accessed 3 January 2019).

Carey, P (2013)
Student as Co-Producer in a Marketised Higher Education System: A Case Study of Students' Experience of Participation in Curriculum Design. *Innovations in Education and Teaching International*, 50(3): 250–60.

Cole, J S (2017)
Concluding Comments about Student Transition to Higher Education. *Higher Education: The International Journal of Higher Education Research*, 73: 539–51.

Coleman, N, Sykes, W and Groom, C (2017)
Peer Support and Children and Young People's Mental Health: Research Review. Department for Education.

Coley, R, Lockwood, D and O'Meara, A (2012)
Deleuze and Guattari and Photography Education. *Rhizome*, 23. [online] Available at: http://rhizomes.net/issue23/coley/index.html (accessed 3 January 2019).

Colley, H (2007)
Understanding Time in Learning Transitions through the Lifecourse. *International Studies in Sociology of Education*, 17(4): 427–43.

Dobinson-Harrington, A (2006)
Personal Tutor Encounters: Understanding the Experience. *Nursing Standard*, 20(50): 35–42.

Ecclestone, K (2009)
Lost and Found in Transition. In Field, J, Gallacher, J and Ingram, R (eds), *Researching Transitions in Lifelong Learning* (pp 9–27). London and New York: Routledge.

Ecclestone, K, Biesta, G and Hughes, M (2010)

Transitions in the Lifecourse: The Role of Identity, Agency and Structure. In Ecclestone, K, Biesta, G and Hughes, M (eds) *Transitions and Learning through the Lifecourse* (pp 1–15). London: Routledge.

Edvardsson Stiwne, E and Jungert, T (2010)

Engineering Students' Experiences of Transition from Study to Work. *Journal of Education and Work*, 23(5): 417–37.

Ellis, S J (2009)

Diversity and Inclusivity at University: A Survey of the Experiences of Lesbian, Gay, Bisexual and Trans (LGBT) Students in the UK. *Higher Education*, 57(6): 723–39.

Epstein, D, O'Flynn, S and Telford, D (2003)

Silenced Sexualities in Schools and Universities. Stoke-on-Trent: Trentham Books.

Equality Challenge Unit (ECU) (2014)

Understanding Adjustments: Supporting Staff and Students who are Experiencing Mental Health Difficulties. [online] Available at: www.ecu. ac.uk/wp-content/uploads/2015/02/ECU_Understanding-adjustments.pdf (accessed 9 January 2019).

Fabri, M, Andrews, P C S and Pukki, H K (2013)

Best Practice for HEI Managers and Senior Academics. [online] Available at: www.plymouth.ac.uk/uploads/production/document/path/10/10863/Best_Practice_Guide_01_screen.pdf (accessed 3 January 2019).

Field, J (2010)

Preface. In Ecclestone, K, Biesta, G and Hughes, M (eds), *Transitions and Learning through the Lifecourse* (pp xvii–xxiv). London: Routledge.

Finnegan, F and Merrill, B (2015)

'We're as Good as Anybody Else': A Comparative Study of Working-Class University Students' Experiences in England and Ireland. *British Journal of Sociology and Education*, 38(3): 307–24.

Formby, E (2012)

Solidarity But Not Similarity? LGBT Communities in the Twenty-First Century. Sheffield: Sheffield Hallam University.

Formby, E (2013)

Understanding and Responding to Homophobia and Bullying: Contrasting Staff and Young People's Views within Community Settings in England. *Sexuality Research and Social Policy*, 10(4): 302–16.

Formby, E (2014)
The Impact of Homophobic and Transphobic Bullying on Education and Employment: A European Survey. Brussels: IGLYO.

Formby, E (2015)
The Limitations of Focussing on Homophobic, Biphobic and Transphobic 'Bullying' to Understand and Address LGBT Young People's Experiences within and Beyond School. Sex Education: Sexuality, Society and Learning, 15(6): 626–40.

Furlong, A (2009)
Revisiting Transitional Metaphors: Reproducing Social Inequalities Under the Conditions of Late Modernity. Journal of Education and Work, 22(5): 343–53.

Gale, T and Parker, S (2014)
Navigating Change: A Typology of Student Transition in Higher Education. Studies in Higher Education, 39(5): 734–53.

Ghenghesh, P (2018)
Personal Tutoring from the Perspectives of Tutors and Tutees. Journal of Further and Higher Education, 42(4): 570–84.

Gibbs, G (2010)
Dimensions of Quality. York: HEA.

Giddens, A (1990)
The Consequences of Modernity. Stanford, CA: Stanford University Press.

Gill, B L, Koch, J, Dlugon, E, Andrew, S and Salamonson, Y (2011)
A Standardised Orientation Program for First Year Undergraduate Students in the College of Health and Science at UWS. A Practice Report. International Journal of the First Year in Higher Education, 2(1): 63–9.

Gubby, L and McNab, N (2013)
Personal Tutoring from the Perspective of the Tutor. Capture 4(1): 7–18.

Harley, D, Winn, S, Pemberton, S and Wilcox, P (2007)
Using Texting to Support Students' Transition to University. Innovations in Education and Teaching International, 44(3): 229–41.

Heirdsfield, A M, Walker, S, Walsh, K and Wilss, L (2008)
Peer Mentoring for First-Year Teacher Education Students: The Mentors' Experience. Mentoring and Tutoring, 16(2): 109–24.

Hillman, K (2005)

The First Year Experience: The Transition from Secondary School to University and TAFE in Australia. Camberwell, VIC: Australian Council for Education Research.

Houlston, C and Smith, P (2009)

The Impact of a Peer Counselling Scheme in an All-Girl Secondary School. *British Journal of Educational Psychology*, 79: 69–86.

Hultberg, J, Plos, K, Hendry, G D and Kjellgren, K I (2009)

Scaffolding Students' Transition to Higher Education: Parallel Introductory Courses for Students and Teachers. *Journal of Further and Higher Education*, 32(1): 47–57.

Ibrahim, A, Kelly, S, Adams, C and Glazebrook, C (2012)

A Systematic Review of Studies of Depression Prevalence in University Students. *Journal of Psychiatric Research*, 47: 391–400.

Ingram, R, Field, J and Gallacher, J (2009)

Learning Transitions: Research, Policy, Practice. In Field, J, Gallacher, J and Ingram, R (eds) *Researching Transitions in Lifelong Learning* (pp 1–6). London and New York: Routledge.

Jamelske, E (2009)

Measuring the Impact of a University First-Year Experience Program on Student GPA and Retention. *Higher Education*, 57(3): 373–91.

James, A (2011)

The Use and Impact of Peer Support Schemes in Schools in the UK, and a Comparison with use in Japan and South Korea. Goldsmiths, University of London.

Kantanis, T (2000)

The Role of Social Transition in Students' Adjustment to the First-Year of University. *Journal of Institutional Research*, 9: 100–10.

Keenan, M (2014)

Coming Out and Fitting In: A Qualitative Exploration of Lesbian, Gay, Bisexual, Trans and Queer Students' University Experiences. Nottingham: Nottingham Trent University.

Kember, D (2001)

Beliefs about Knowledge and the Process of Teaching and Learning as a Factor in Adjusting to Study in Higher Education. *Studies in Higher Education*, 26(2): 205–21.

Kift, S (2009)

Articulating a Transition Pedagogy to Scaffold and to Enhance the First Year Student Learning Experience in Australian Higher Education: Final Report for ALTC Senior Fellowship Program. Strawberry Hills, NSW: Australian Learning and Teaching Council.

Kift, S and Nelson, K (2005)

Beyond Curriculum Reform: Embedding the Transition Experience. Paper presented at the Higher Education Research and Development Society of Australasia (HERDSA) conference, Higher Education in a Changing World, 225–35. http://conference.herdsa.org.au/2005/pdf/refereed/paper_294.pdf (accessed 3 January 2019).

Kift, S, Nelson, K and Clarke, J (2010)

Transition Pedagogy: A Third Generation Approach to FYE: A Case Study of Policy and Practice for the Higher Education Sector. *International Journal of the First Year in Higher Education*, 1(1): 1–20.

Krause, K (2005)

The Changing Face of the First Year: Challenges for Policy and Practice in Research-Led Universities. Keynote paper at the University of Queensland First Year Experience Workshop, October.

Krause, K-L and Coates, H (2008)

Students' Engagement in First-Year University. *Assessment and Evaluation in Higher Education*, 33(5): 493–505.

Leese, M (2010)

Bridging the Gap: Supporting Student Transitions into Higher Education. *Journal of Further and Higher Education*, 34(2): 239–51.

Lemanski, T, Mewis, R and Overton, T (2011)

An Introduction to Work-Based Learning: A Physical Sciences Practice Guide. [online] Available at: www.heacademy.ac.uk/system/files/work_based_learning.pdf (accessed 9 January 2019).

Lent, R W, Nota, L, Soresi, S and Ferrari, L (2007)

Realistic Major Previews in the School-to-College Transition of Italian High School Students. *Career Development Quarterly*, 56(2): 183–91.

MBF (2011)

Peer Mentoring in Schools: A Review of the Evidence Base of the Benefits of Peer Mentoring in Schools Including Findings from the MBF Outcomes Measurement Programme, 2010. Manchester: Mentoring and Befriending Foundation.

McCulloch, A (2009)
The Student as Co-Producer: Learning from Public Administration about the Student–University Relationship. *Studies in Higher Education*, 34: 171–83.

McKinney, J S (2005)
On the Margins: A Study of the Experiences of Transgender College Students. *Journal of Gay and Lesbian Issues in Education*, 3(1): 63–76.

Meehan, C and Howells, K (2018)
'What Really Matters to Freshers?' Evaluation of First Year Student Experience of Transition into University. *Journal of Further and Higher Education*, 42(7): 893–907.

Metcalfe, J, Wilson, S and Levecque, K (2018)
Exploring Wellbeing and Mental Health and Associated Support Services for Postgraduate Researchers. Cambridge: Vitae.

Metro (2014)
Youth Chances Survey of 16–25 Year Olds: First Reference Report. London: Metro.

Mitchall, A and Jaeger, A (2018)
Parental Influences on Low-Income, First-Generation Students' Motivation on the Path to College. *Journal of Higher Education*, 89(4): 582–609.

Molesworth, M, Nixon, E and Scullion, R (2009)
Having, Being and Higher Education: The Marketisation of the University and the Transformation of the Student into Consumer. *Teaching in Higher Education*, 14: 277–87.

Morrow, J and Ackermann, M (2012)
Intention to Persist and Retention of First-Year Students: The Importance of Motivation and Sense of Belonging. *College Student Journal*, 46: 483–91.

Neary, M (2010)
Student as Producer: A Pedagogy for the Avant-Garde? *Learning Exchange*, 1(1). [online] Available at: http://studentasproducer.lincoln.ac.uk/files/2014/03/15-72-1-pb-1.pdf (accessed 13 February 2019).

Neary, M (2012)
Student as Producer: An Institution of the Common? [Or How to Recover Communist/Revolutionary Science]. *Journal of Enhancing Learning in the Social Sciences*, 4(3): 1–16.

NUS (2014)
Education Beyond the Straight and Narrow: LGBT Students' Experience in Higher Education. London: NUS.

O'Leary, S (2016)
The Opportunities and Challenges for Employability-Related Support in STEM Degrees. *New Directions in the Teaching of Physical Sciences*, 11(4): 1–11.

Osborne, M and Gallacher, J (2007)
An International Perspective on Researching Widening Access. In Osborne, M, Gallacher, J and Crossan, B (eds) *Researching Widening Access to Lifelong Learning: Issues and Approaches in International Research* (pp 3–16). London: Routledge.

Pallas, A M (2003)
Educational Transitions, Trajectories, and Pathways. In Mortimer, J T and Shanahan, M J (eds) *Handbook of the Life Course* (pp 165–84). New York: Plenum.

Parkinson, G and Forrester, G (2004)
'Mind the Gap': Students' Expectations and Perceptions of Induction to Distance Learning in Higher Education. Paper presented at the British Educational Research Association Annual Conference, University of Manchester. [online] Available at: www.leeds.ac.uk/educol/documents/00003842.doc (accessed 3 January 2019).

Potts, E (2017)
The Relationship between Campus Climate, Perceived Stigma, Perceived Social Support, and Students' Decisions to Disclose their Mental Health-Problems on Campus. Philadelphia College of Osteopathic Medicine.

Price, M, Rust, C, O'Donovan, B, Hindley, K and Bryant, R (2012)
Assessment Literacy: The Foundation for Improving Student Learning. Oxford: Oxford Centre for Staff and Learning Development.

Quinn, J (2010)
Rethinking 'Failed Transitions' to Higher Education. In Ecclestone, K, Biesta, G and Hughes, M (eds) *Transitions and Learning through the Lifecourse* (pp 118–29). London: Routledge.

Reason, R (2009)
Student Variables that Predict Retention: Recent Research and New Developments. *NASPA Journal*, 46: 482–501.

Reay, D, David, M and Ball, S (2005)
Degrees of Choice: Social Class, Race and Gender in Higher Education. Stoke-on-Trent: Trentham Books.

Ribchester, C, Ross, K and Rees, E (2014)

Examining the Impact of Pre-Induction Social Networking on the Student Transition into Higher Education. *Journal of Innovations in Education and Teaching International*, 51(4): 355–65.

Ross, J, Head, K, King, L, Perry, P M and Smith, S (2014)

The Personal Development Tutor Role: An Exploration of Student and Lecturer Experiences and Perceptions of That Relationship. *Nurse Education Today*, 34(9): 1207–13.

Saunders, D B (2011)

Students as Customers: The Influence of Neoliberal Ideology and Free-Market Logic on Entering First-Year College Students. *Open Access Dissertations*, paper 377. [online] Available at: http://scholarworks.umass.edu/open_access_dissertations/377 (accessed 3 January 2019).

Scanlon, L, Rowling, L and Weber, Z (2007)

'You Don't Have Like an Identity… You Are Just Lost in a Crowd': Forming a Student Identity in the First-Year Transition to University. *Journal of Youth Studies*, 10(2): 223–41.

Schreiner, L, Patrice, N, Anderson, E and Cantwell, L (2011)

The Impact of Faculty and Staff on High-Risk College Student Persistence. *Journal of College Student Development*, 52: 321–38.

Sellar, S and Gale, T (2011)

Mobility, Aspiration, Voice: A New Structure of Feeling for Student Equity in Higher Education. *Critical Studies in Education*, 52(2): 115–34.

Smith, D I (2009)

Changes in Transitions: The Role of Mobility, Class and Gender. *Journal of Education and Work*, 22(5): 369–90.

Stephen, D E, O'Connell, P and Hall, M (2008)

'Going the Extra Mile', 'Fire-Fighting', or 'Laissez-Faire'? Re-Evaluating Personal Tutoring Relationships within Mass Higher Education. *Teaching in Higher Education*, 13(4): 449–60.

Taulke-Johnson, R (2010)

Queer Decisions? Gay Male Students' University Choices. *Studies in Higher Education*, 35(3): 247–61.

Thomas, L (2002)

Student Retention in Higher Education: The Role of Institutional Habitus. *Journal of Education Policy*, 17(4): 423–42.

Trautwein, C and Bosse, E (2017)

The First Year in Higher Education: Critical Requirements from the Student Perspective. *Higher Education: The International Journal of Higher Education Research*, 73: 371–87.

Universities UK and Papyrus (2014)

Suicide-Safer Universities. [online] Available at: www.universitiesuk.ac.uk/policy-and-analysis/reports/Pages/guidance-for-universities-on-preventing-student-suicides.aspx (accessed 3 January 2019).

Valentine, G, Skelton, T and Butler, R (2003)

Coming Out and Outcomes: Negotiating Lesbian and Gay Identities with, and in, the Family. *Environment and Planning D: Society and Space*, 21(4): 479–99.

Valentine, G, Wood, N and Plummer, P (2009)

The Experience of Lesbian, Gay, Bisexual and Trans Staff and Students in Higher Education. London: Equality Challenge Unit.

Weare, K and Nind, M (2011)

Mental Health Promotion and Problem Prevention in Schools: What Does the Evidence Say? *Health Promotion International*, 26(1): 29–69.

Weeks, J, Heaphy, B and Donovan, C (2001)

Same Sex Intimacies: Families of Choice and Other Life Experiments. London: Routledge.

Wellington, J and Sikes, P (2006)

'A Doctorate in a Tight Compartment': Why Do Students Choose a Professional Doctorate and What Impact Does it Have on Their Personal and Professional Lives? *Studies in Higher Education*, 31(6): 723–34.

Werner, H (1957)

The Concept of Development from a Comparative and Organismic Point of View. In Harris, D B (ed) *The Concept of Development: An Issue in the Study of Human Behaviour* (pp 125–48). Minneapolis: University of Minnesota Press.

Winn, S (2002)

Student Motivations: A Socio-Economic Perspective. *Studies in Higher Education*, 27(4): 445–57.

Woodall, T, Hiller, A and Resnick, S (2012)

Making Sense of Higher Education: Students as Consumers and the Value of the University Experience. *Studies in Higher Education*, 1–20.

Wootton, S (2013)
Personal Tutoring for the 21st Century, Further Education Tutorial Network (FETN). [online] Available at: https://api.excellencegateway.org.uk/resource/eg:6301 (accessed 3 January 2019).

World Health Organization (WHO) (2014)
Mental Health: A State of Well-Being. [online] Available at: www.who.int/features/factfiles/mental_health/en (accessed 7 January 2019).

Worth, N (2009)
Understanding Youth Transition as 'Becoming': Identity, Time and Futurity. *Geoforum*, 40(6): 1050–60.

+INDEX

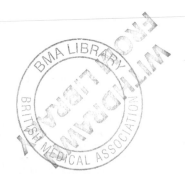